P9-CAM-314

The POCKET COMPANION OF NONPRESCRIPTION MEDICATIONS, First Edition, attempts to present the most common trade or brand names and adult doses, and should be used only as a guideline to these; it should not be considered as an official therapeutic document. If there is a discrepancy in therapeutic class, preparations, and dosages, the reader is advised to obtain official and more complete information from the pharmaceutical manufacturer and/or package insert.

The Author or Publisher are not responsible for typographical errors within the contents of this guide.

ISBN: 0-9677721-1-7

Published by Global Publishing Network
P.O. Box 850439
New Orleans, LA 70185-0439

Phone: (504) 779-0383: Fax: (504) 779-0383
E-Mail: AAruna@aol.com OR Amazon.com
Website: http://vsp.wpg.net/JN/GLOBALPUBLISHING

Indexer — Mary E. Coe
(301) 279-9317

Cover design by Graphics Color Solutions, Inc., New Orleans, LA

Printed in the United States of America

NONPRESCRIPTION (OTC) MEDICATIONS:

COUNSELING GUIDELINES ON
THE SAFE USE OF OVER-THE-COUNTER MEDICINES.

First Edition

A POCKET COMPANION FOR
PHARMACISTS, PHARMACY STUDENTS, PHYSICIANS, ALLIED HEALTH
PRACTITIONERS AND CONSUMERS

Augustine S. Aruna, Pharm.D.,FASCP
Associate Professor of Clinical Pharmacy
Xavier University of Louisiana College of Pharmacy
New Orleans, Louisiana 70125
and
Clinical Pharmacy Consultant
Department of Veterans Affairs Medical Center
New Orleans, Louisiana 70146

FOREWORD

Currently available references in the realm of nonprescription products tend to go deeper into background information than the lay public can understand, or are poorly organized for quick yet scholarly reference. In this book Dr. Aruna has compiled in easy to use tabular form the various classes of nonprescription drugs, but with a clear emphasis on the counseling information that should accompany the use of these products. For the consumer who purchases his or her nonprescription products from a non-pharmacy source, or under circumstances where there is no contact with a health professional, this reference is a quick counseling guide. Dr. Aruna has made the information concise and easy to find, but has also been unabashed in stating when such products should NOT be used, rather than leaving a vague judgement call in the hands of a lay reader. In this sense this text is very useful for the layman.

The reference also includes tables dealing with areas that other layman-intended texts on the subject often shy away from such as personal care products, ostomy products, enteral feeding products, herbal and phytomedicinal products, and medical and health supplies. This has been a gap in many publications dealing with nonprescription products, as these items are not considered drugs by many who are writing such texts. Such information is deemed inappropriate. In this sense, Dr. Aruna's material is more real world in its acceptance of patient/consumer needs and experience.

For the student, Dr. Aruna has made a study text available that serves to categorize and organize the wide variety of information about nonprescription products without encumbering it with the dense background and prerequisite knowledge from pharmacology, pharmacokinetics, pathophysiology, etc., which students might be expected to bring to a formal course of instruction. For the student as with the layperson, the emphasis should be on what advice or counsel that should be given to the patient, and this text summarizes this information nicely. For the student, the reference also helps them to prepare for the national pharmacy licensure examination known as NAPLEX. It identifies for the student the competencies expected to be mastered for this examination and provides sample questions of the type that might appear on the examination. It is an excellent study and examination preparation guide for students. For the practitioner and health professional the reference is quick and easy to use, and because of its size, easy to carry about to be used as needed.

Victor A. Padron, Ph.D.
Associate Professor of Pharmacy Practice
Creighton University
School of Pharmacy and Allied Health Professions
Omaha, Nebraska 68178

PREFACE

Many patients self-medicate with over-the-counter (OTC) medications without seeking the advice of a pharmacist. The problem with this is that some OTC medications can interact with other drugs the patient may be taking or can exacerbate a pre-existing disease or condition. One of the leading causes of therapeutic outcome failure is drug noncompliance resulting from the co-administration of OTC medications. Medications have little or no chance of therapeutic success if they are not taken properly. The answer to this serious problem involves adequate patient counseling. Adequate patient counseling by the pharmacist can encourage good drug regimen compliance and maximize therapeutic outcome.

The algorithm(s) and tables outlined in this book provide counseling guidelines on OTC medications. The tables outline various conditions, treatment modalities, side-effects associated with treatment, and disease states in which treatment should be avoided or in which an alternate form of therapy should be initiated. Proper use of these tables prior to self-medication can improve therapeutic outcomes, decrease noncompliance, increase awareness of side effects and alleviate many problems.

This book also contains invaluable highlights on the National Association of Boards of Pharmacy Licensure Examination (NABPLEX) which has recently become the North American Pharmacy Licensing Examination (NAPLEX) and integrates pharmacy practice competencies existing in the U.S. and Canada. It provides the student preparing for NAPLEX with the OTC component which comprises 25% of the examination. A series of sample questions and a key are provided to facilitate preparation for the examination. The pocket book also presents the NAPLEX Competency Statements pertaining to the OTC portion of the test for quick reference.

The last section of the book contains sample practical clinical scenarios for students and practitioners to use in developing problem-based learning skills and in applying their theoretical knowledge of nonprescription drug therapeutics. These practical assessment techniques will help them collect and synthesize factual information; analyze that information and apply it to prevent a problem from occurring or to formulate a rational solution.

Augustine S. Aruna,Pharm.D.,FASCP

4

4.00.00

MONITORING DRUG THERAPY

(25% of total test)

OTC Component

4.02.00   **Given a medical history, medication record, drug therapy history, or a set of prescriptions or medication orders, the candidate shall identify or remedy interactions or contraindications involving prescription or OTC products in drug therapy, including those with other drugs.**

01.   The candidate shall identify or remedy interactions or contraindications with disease states or medical conditions.

02.   The candidate shall identify or remedy interactions or contraindications with diagnostic tests or procedures.

03.   The candidate shall identify or remedy interactions or contraindications with sensitivities or allergies; genetic, environmental or biosocial factors (e.g., geriatric, pediatric, pregnant, post-surgical, ileostomy).

04.   The candidate shall identify or remedy interactions or contraindications with special diets or dietary practices.

5.00.00
Counseling Patients and Health Professionals
(25% of total test)

OTC Component

5.04.00   **The candidate shall identify the name, correct therapeutic classification, pharmacological action, ingredients, physical description or dosage form, or drug release mechanism of OTC drugs.**

01. The candidate shall determine whether a given drug is obtainable by OTC purchase.

5.05.00   The candidate shall advise consumers regarding the selection, proper use, effects, precautions, or contraindications of OTC drugs.

01. The candidate shall determine whether a patient's condition requires medical supervision or self-medication.

02. The candidate shall explain an OTC drug's action in terms that consumers are likely to understand.

03. The candidate shall explain how an OTC drug shall be taken (e.g., dosage, time of day, frequency, before or after meals).

04. The candidate shall provide proper auxiliary instructions for an OTC medication.

05. The candidate shall provide the recommended duration of use for an OTC medication.

06. The candidate shall explain appropriate cautions for use of an OTC medication by members of special patient populations (e.g., diabetic, asthmatic, hypertensive, geriatric, pediatric).

07. The candidate shall explain the major factors related to drug stability or proper storage of an OTC medication.

08. The candidate shall identify situations requiring medical advice if an OTC medication causes an untoward or inadequate effect.

5.06.00   The candidate shall recognize the use of medical/surgical appliances or devices, durable medical equipment, or prescription accessories or shall counsel regarding the selection, use, or storage of such items (e.g., thermometers; ostomy appliances; contraceptives; catheters; needles, syringes, or diabetic supplies; diagnostic products; contact lens preparations).

5.07.00   The candidate shall identify or explain contemporary public health issues or principles of nutrition in relation to the treatment of diseases or medical or physiologic conditions.
[OTC, Nutrition & Pharmacy Practice Courses]

01.   The candidate shall identify or describe approved and accepted nutritional requirements or demonstrate knowledge of nutrition-related topics, including:
   a.   Common disease conditions or symptoms caused by vitamin or mineral deficiencies or excessive use;
   b.   Natural sources of vitamins or minerals;
   c.   Nonessential ingredients of nutritional supplements; or
   d.   potential untoward effects of nutrients, foods, food components, or food additives on the development or course of diseases or sensitivities.

02.   The candidate shall apply biochemical principles of nutrition in relation to special patient populations or treatments, including:
   a.   Prenatal or postnatal care;
   b.   Pediatric, adult, or geriatric nutritional requirements or formulas; or
   c.   Enteral therapy, parenteral therapy or formulas.

03.   The candidate shall identify or explain procedures other than drug and nutritional therapy that are effective in preventing or minimizing the progress of diseases (e.g., herpes, AIDS, cancer, chemical dependency, cardiovascular disease, sexually transmitted disease).

TABLE OF CONTENTS

FEATURES IN NONPRESCRIPTION DRUGS AND PRODUCTS

Subject Description	Subject Rationale
a. Familiarization with OTC medications and products. b. Focus on pharmacology of OTC agents. c. Discussion of disease states involving OTC drug use. d. Discussion of self-medication. e. Discussion of drug product selection (DPS). f. Emphasis on patient counseling with respect to OTC agents.	a. The pharmacist is the most accessible health care practitioner. b. Consequently, good knowledge of OTC medications and products, pathophysiology of common diseases, proper use of drugs and devices and good communication and ethical skills are of paramount importance in patient assessment and DPS. c. Accurate patient assessment determines the outcome.

NAPLEX Competency	Objectives
a. OTC drugs and products constitute about 25% of NAPLEX. b. Hence, contribution of OTC to success on the examination cannot be overemphasized.	a. Emphasize pharmacology, indications, contraindications (e.g., aspirin in asthma), adverse drug reactions (ADRs), safe dosage ranges, interactions (e.g., aspirin with warfarin, cimetidine with theophylline). b. Emphasize the ability to make rationale DPS based on comparative safety/efficacy profiles, especially for special populations (e.g., elderly, women, children, renally and/or hepatically compromised patients). c. Emphasize counseling skills with respect to OTC drugs/products (e.g., appropriate dose, route of drug administration, duration of action of drug, ADRs, interactions, precautionary measures). d. Recognition of indicators for patient referrals to physicians and other agencies).

Background	Background
a. OTC drugs are medicines purchased without written prescription for symptomatic relief of self-limiting conditions (e.g., stomach indigestion, headache, upper respiratory tract complaints, minor skin problems-cuts, burns, dandruff). b. There are hundreds to thousands of OTC products on the market. c. OTC products expenditure is approximately $14.2 billion per annum. The projection is $34 billion by year 2000.	d. Average cost of OTC drugs/yr/adult is $47. e. Average prescription drug cost in 1992 was $24. f. Considerations: - margin of safety - label information - methods of promotion - methods of distribution

Adapted from The Handbook of Nonprescription Drugs (APhA), 11th Edition 1996;References 1-10, page 14.

FDA OTC Drug Review Advisory Panels of Scientists	FDA Categorization of OTC Drug Ingredients
a. Purpose is to ensure safety, efficacy, proper labeling of ingredients in OTC products.	I. Safe and effective for claimed therapeutic indication.
b. Review process is expensive and is supported by both government and pharmaceutical industry.	II. Not generally safe and effective or unacceptable indications.
	III. Insufficient data available to permit final classification in either category I or II.

FDA Classes of Drug Recalls (Voluntary removal of drugs from the market following drug-induced health threats or safety)	Consumer Practices & Demographics
I. Due to serious or fatal consequences II. Due to serious and irreversible sequelae III. Due to products not likely to cause serious but some minor adverse drug reactions.	a. Supermarkets sell 40% of OTC products. b. Supermarkets sell 20% of recent prescription to OTC drugs. c. Sixty percent (60%) of OTC drugs are sold in retail and community pharmacies.

Consumer Practices & Demographics: Geriatrics	Consumer Practices & Demographics: Women
a. Fastest growing segment of US population (12.5%). b. Purchases 35% of OTC drugs. c. Consumption likely to rise to 50% by year 2000. d. About 87% will use drugs improperly.	a. Purchase more OTC products than men because most of their needs cost more. b. Evolution of women in the work force has led to development of anxiety, skin disorders, stomach indigestion, weight complaints and general well-being.

Consumer Practices & Demographics:	Consumer Practices & Demographics:
Men	**Children**
Most likely to purchase OTC medications for overworked muscles, minor cuts and scratches.	Frequently require OTC drugs for allergy and common colds, analgesics and antipyretics.

Drug Information Resources for Consumers	Consumer Education

a. Health professionals (e.g., pharmacists, nurses, physicians).
b. Advertisements:
   - Print media (e.g., books, magazines, newspapers, PDR).
   - Broadcast media (e.g., radio, TV).
c. Friends.
d. Relatives.
	a. Highly educated individuals are more likely to purchase OTC medications recommended by pharmacists and are more likely to follow directions than less educated persons.
	b. Other factors affecting consumption:
	   - age and socioeconomic status.
	   - trust and reputation of pharmacists and pharmacies.
	   - quick and reliable service.

Factors Influencing OTC Counseling	Readability of OTC Labels (Contents)
a. Financial reimbursement. b. Need more time. c. Pharmacists need more informational/educational aids. d. Specific areas in pharmacy dedicated to patient counseling.	a. Product identification - active/inactive ingredients. b. Name of manufacturer, distributor or packer. c. Directions for use; amount, route, dosing. d. Warnings; side effects, contraindications. e. Label "Flags"; any new revision or change. f. Precautions; significant drug/food interactions. g. "Keep Out of Reach of Children" warning. h. OTC products sold in tamper-resistant packaging (TRP) to prevent criminal tampering (e.g., Tylenol tampering case). i. Alcohol-containing products (> 5%) in child-resistant closures to avoid accidental ingestion. j. Expiration date.

FDA Criteria for Prescription to OTC status Switch	Advantages of Prescription to OTC Switch
a. Proven safety. b. Limited risks. c. Proven efficacy. d. Simple instructions.	a. Consumer savings. b. Reduction in costly prescription drug prescribing. c. Higher manufacturer profit index. d. Convenience and wider outlet of distribution. e. Expanded opportunities for self-care and self.medication. f. Expanded pharmacists counseling demands.

13

Disadvantages of Prescription to OTC Switch	Proposal for Third Class of Drugs
a. Limited availability for Medicaid recipients. b. Potential health risk to uneducated or uninformed consumers. c. More pharmacist counseling demands. d. Increase in legal liability.	a. Currently 2 classes of drugs: Prescription and Nonprescription. b. Prescription drugs are controlled mostly by physicians and pharmacists. c. There has been a proposal to create a third class of drugs called "Pharmacist Legend" or "Transitional Class" or "Restrictive Sales" dispensed and sold exclusively by pharmacists. d. The Food and Drug Administration (FDA), American Medical Association (AMA) and Nonprescription drug Manufacturers Association (NDMA) are opposed to the idea.

Disadvantages of Third Class of Drugs	Advantages of Third Class of Drugs
a. No such thing as a half-safe drug. b. Expansion of legal liability. c. A form of pharmacist prescribing! Note that clinical pharmacists with advanced training now have limited prescribing authority of legend drugs!!!	a. Saves patient time and expense from physician visit. b. Prevents misuse of the drugs. c. Provides a market window to evaluate potential prescription-to-OTC drugs.

Generic Drugs	Criteria for Approval of Generic Drugs
a. FDA-approved drugs have 2 names-Generic and Brand. b. A generic drug is a chemical compound of active ingredient(s). c. A brand name is the trade name selected by the manufacturer that markets the drug. d. The manufacturer has the patent (legal and exclusive rights to sell the drug by its brand name) for 17 years. e. Upon expiration of the patent, competitive manufacturers can market the generic drug or use another brand name. f. Generic drugs must undergo FDA approval process, but no duplication of clinical studies is required. Generic houses must comply with rigid standards set by the NDMA.	a. Safety and efficacy. b. Bioequivalence and therapeutic equivalence. c. The generic and brand drugs generally have similar bioavailability.

Reasons for Growth of Generics Market	Ten Top Generic Drug Companies
a Large number of drugs coming off patent. b. Enforced and stream-lined FDA approval process (no additional clinical trials required). c. About 200 generics approved per year. d. Health Care Reform: Cost-containment efforts from insurance companies forcing consumers to spend more on generics.	a. Apothecon b. Rugby Laboratories c. Boots Pharmaceuticals d. Goldline Laboratories e. Geneva Pharmaceuticals f. Mylan Pharmaceuticals g. Schein Pharmaceuticals h. Major Pharmaceuticals I. Barr Laboratories j. Warner-Chilcott

OTC Medications During Pregnancy and Lactation	Factors to Consider with respect to Drugs and Fetal Harm
a. Most feared questions encountered by pharmacists involves medication use during pregnancy and lactation. b. Teratogenic effects will lead to noncompliance during pregnancy. c. Temporary use of some OTC agents may not be harmful. d. Consider use of other causes of teratogenicity such as tobacco, alcohol, caffeine in beverages, environmental hazards (pollution, fumes, chemicals), factors which must be ruled-out. e. Drug-related birth defects may not appear for months or years after birth.	a. Lack of certain nutrients (e.g., Neural Tube Defect (NTD) secondary to folic acid deficiency). b. Type of medication. c. Amount of drug ingested. d. Length of time the medicine is taken. e. Stage of pregnancy (trimesters).

Some OTC Drugs that are Safe in Pregnancy

a. Acetaminophen (APAP) [Tylenol]
b. Antacids (Aluminum/magnesium/calcium-containing antacids)
c. Antihistamines such as Chlorpheniramine [Chlortrimeton] and diphenhydramine [Benadryl].
   Note: Anticholinergic effects associated with antihistamines may cause inhibition of lactation.
d. Decongestants such as pseudoephedrine [Sudafed] - best in last 2 trimesters.
e. Laxatives such as stool softeners, docusate potassium or docusate calcium [Surfak] (versus docusate sodium [Colace] and docusate sodium+casanthranol [Peri-colace]) and bulk laxatives (e.g., psyllium [Metamucil]) are preferred during pregnancy and lactation.

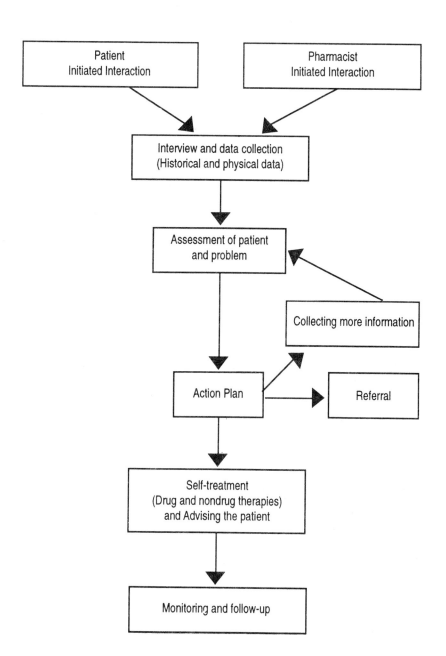

Flow Chart 1. Patient - Pharmacist consultation process.

Adapted from The Handbook of Nonprescription Drugs (APhA), 11th Edition, 1996;References 1-85, Pages 31-32.

PATIENT-PHARMACIST CONSULTATION PROCESS

Although warnings are required on the labels of OTC products, labeling alone may be inadequate; the patient may often need assistance in selecting and properly using nonprescription drugs. Because inappropriate use and misuse of nonprescritpion drugs can increase the risk of drug misadventures, resulting in increased cost and a more seriously ill patient, the pharmacist's role in counseling and assessment can be crucial.

To serve patients better, pharmacies need to maximize the personal service of the pharmacist. Patient inquiries should always be referred to the pharmacist, who must actively promote the value of a pharmacist's guidance in selecting and monitoring treatment with a nonprescription drug. It is essential to increase the patient's awareness of the importance of consulting the pharmacist, not only when considering a drug for the first time but also when making subsequent purchases.

Patients rank providing nonprescription drug information as a very important pharmacy service. In one study, the majority of patients considered pharmacists to be competent and to have a professional relationship with their patients. The pharmacist is responsible for providing pharmaceutical care which entails designing, implementing, and monitoring a therapeutic plan, in cooperation with the patient and other health professionals, to produce specific therapeutic outcomes. Under this concept, each time a patient presents a therapeutic request (i.e., a question about self-care or drug therapy, a request for a new prescription), the pharmacist systematically works with the patient and other health care providers to identify any actual or potential drug therapy problems and to review and determine the best response to the patient's drug-related needs. This system is referred to as the "comprehensive pharmaceutical care process". Within this process, the pharmacist reviews all the medications that a patient is taking as a prerequisite of assessment and consultation. Drug regimen review considerations include all the medicosocioeconomic issues encompassing drug indications, safety or adverse drug reactions, efficacy or effectiveness, therapeutic outcomes, cost-effectiveness, compliance, drug regimen complexity, and untreated indication or condition.

The goal of each patient encounter is to prevent, detect, and resolve drug therapy problems. To do this, the pharmacist must establish an efficient method of gathering pertinent information so that any such problems can be assessed. Since the single most important piece of information is an accurate accounting of all medications that the patient is currently using, the pharmacist must obtain these data first. Counseling patients involves advising patients on self-treatment which is an important part of pharmacy practice and provides the pharmacist with an opportunity to act in a primary care role. Often the patient's first contact with the health care system, the pharmacist, can assess the situation and recommend a course of action. This may include recommending a nonprescription drug, dissuading the patient from buying medication when drug therapy is not indicated, recommending nondrug treatment, or referring the patient to another health care practitioner. Interventions by pharmacists through consultation and effective educational strategies can enhance patient compliance. Good and effective communication skills are absolutley essential in this process.

Interventions by pharmacists through consultation and effective educational strategies can enhance patient compliance. The goal of this patient-pharmacist interaction is to establish a therapeutic relationship. Good and effective communication skills are absolutely essential in this process. Flow Chart 1 illustrates the patient-pharmacist consultation process which includes the patient interview or information-gathering process, assessment of patient condition, action plan (collecting more information, selecting physician referral), selecting self-treatment and advising the patient on self-treatment, and maintaining follow-up contact. Before formulating a plan for self-treatment or physician referral, the pharmacist must obtain enough information to identify and assess the problem. The most important piece of information the pharmacist must obtain is an accurate accounting of each active medication the patient is using to treat all of his or her medical conditions. Fortunately, within the context of providing comprehensive pharmaceutical care, the pharmacist need not try to obtain all relevant information in one encounter. The follow-up step of care continues the initial assessment process and allows the pharmacist the luxury of obtaining additional information.

Patient interview involves collection of historical or patient-specific data (e.g., medication history, lifestyle, demographic) and physical assessment (e.g., pulse rate, heart sounds, respiratory rate, age, weight) using such techniques as observation or inspection, palpation or manipulations, percussion, and auscultation. Good observational skills are very valuable. Assessment is the evaluation of all the data-historical and physical-collected from the patient to determine the etiology and severity of the medical condition. Determining etiology and severity is essential for reaching appropriate conclusions about treatment and the need for referral. Assessment of severity will vary depending on the problem. In general, the more severe the problem, the greater the potential for referral. After collecting all the available information and assessing the patient's condition, the pharmacist must quickly formulate an action plan. A sound action plan requires paying careful attention to five specific areas including collecting more information, selecting physician referral (e.g., too severe, persistent, recurring or complicated symptoms), selecting self-treatment (e.g., drug, nondrug), advising the patient on self-treatment (e.g., drug dosing, therapeutic and adverse effects, drug interactions, available dosage forms, generic availability, general treatment guidelines including lifestyle changes, additional products or services, informational sources, duration of therapy, etc.), and maintaining follow-up contact for outcomes assessment.

The tables are designed in such a way that OTC information normally covered in a textbook chapter or chapters is summarized on a single page. Column 1 of each table lists the generic and branded names of drugs or products. Columns 2 and/or 3 present additional and pertinent product information and counseling guidelines for quick and easy reference.

Table 1

CENTRAL NERVOUS SYSTEM (CNS) STIMULANTS

Pharmacologic Products	Counseling Guidelines

A. Caffeine   - FDA-approved stimulant
           - Methylxanthine derivative
B. Ephedrine - Not FDA-approved
           - Sympathomimetic
           - DO NOT RECOMMEND!
 	
1. Caffeine 100 mg Chewable Tablets [NoDoz]
2. Caffeine 200 mg Caplets [NoDoz MS]
3. Caffeine 150 mg Tablets [Quick-Pep]
4. Caffeine 200 mg Caplets & Tablets [Vivarin]
5. Caffeine 200 mg, SR Caplets [Caffedrine]
6. 20/20 Tablets 200 mg
7. 357 Magnum II 200 mg Tablets
8. Dexitac Capsules SR 250 mg
9. King of Hearts Tablets 200 mg
10. Overtime Tablets 200 mg
11. Pep-Back Tablets 100 mg
12. Pep-Back Ultra Caplets 200 mg
 	
## Non Pharmacologic Products: 	
 	
1. Coffee
2. Tea
3. Cocoa
4. Chocolate milk
5. Chocolate candy
6. Cola
	Caffeine causes the heart rate to increase especially when it interacts with a sympathomimetic such as phenylpropanolamine or with monoamine oxidase inhibitors.
	
	Caffeine interacts with theophylline to cause an increase in theophylline levels and possible theophylline toxicity.
	
	Caffeine may antagonize the effects of diazepam.
	
	Caffeine may decrease iron absorption.
	
	Caffeine promotes urination - incontinence
	
	Caffeine causes stomach distress especially when it interacts with NSAIDS, aspirin, steroids and alcohol.
	
	Withdrawal effects include sleepiness, increased irritability, and headaches
	
	Do not use stimulant products regularly. They can cause toxicity (caffeinism).
	
	Patients with heart problems or circulatory diseases should get clearance from a physician before taking any stimulant products.

Table 2a

SLEEP AIDS

Sleep Management	Counseling Guidelines
Pharmacologic Management of insomnia Antihistamines : **Diphenhydramine HCL 25 mg caps** [Benadryl, Nytol, Sleep-eze 3, Sominex, Sominex Pain Relief (500-650 mg APAP), Nervine, SleepWell 2-nite, Bayer Select MS (500-650 mg APAP)]. **Diphenhydramine HCL 50 mg caps** [MS Nytol, Sominex Caplets, Nighttime Pamprin (500-650 mg APAP), MS Unisom, Unisom w/Pain Relief 500-650 mg APAP)] **Diphenhydramine Citrate 38 mg Caplets** [Bufferin AF Nite Time Caplets (+ 500 mg APAP)] **Chlorpheniramine maleate 4 mg, 8 mg, 8 mg SR, 12 mg, 12 mg SR tablets** [Tranquil,Chlortrimeton] **Pyrilamine maleate 25 mg tablets** [Somnicaps] **Doxylamine succinate 25 mg tablets** [Unisom]	1. Do not give to children under 12 (anticholinergic toxicity). 2. If sleepiness persists continuously for more than two weeks, consult a doctor. 3. Do not take this product if there is asthma, glaucoma, emphysema, chronic pulmonary disease, shortness of breath, or difficulty in urination (e.g., due to prostatic hypertrophy). 4. Avoid alcoholic beverages while taking this product (oversedation). 5. Avoid driving an automobile or operating hazardous machinery (sedation/blurred vision). 6. Tricyclic antidepressants (TCAs)/anticholinergics + sleep aid will cause synergism (more sleep). 7. Consult pharmacist if you experience adverse effects including dizziness, ringing in ears (tinnitus), blurred vision, nervousness, heart palpitations, increased irritability, and hallucinations.

SLEEP AIDS

Sleep Management	Counseling Guidelines
Miscellaneous Products 1. L-Tryptophan 1-3 gm 2. Valerian 405 mg PO tid 3. Melatonin 0.1-1 mg qhs 4. Alcohol (Ethanol) **Non-Pharmacologic Management** Walk around for awhile - get tired. Try watching television or reading. Drink a glass of warm milk. Avoid large meals at bedtime. Soak in a tub of warm water.	8. Avoid L-Tryptophan use as sleep aid. Efficacy is questionable. More than 1,500 cases of eosinophilia-myalgia syndrome(EMS) including at least 27 deaths reported. Interaction between L-Tryptophan and MAOIs resulting in "serotonin storm" (symptoms include agitation, restlessness, aggressiveness, tremor, hyperthermia, diarrhea, and cramping) reported. Not recommended for insomnia. 9. Valerian (derived from the plant Valeriana officinalis) is a "traditional herbal remedy" for sleep induction. 10. Melatonin (endogenous hormone produced by pineal gland). Sleep-inducing effects largely unknown. 11. Alcohol (CNS depressant/sedative) sleep-inducing efficacy data limited. Alone or in combination with acetaminophen can cause liver injury. Avoid with other CNS depressants, including benzodiazepines.

WEIGHT AND DIET CONTROL PRODUCTS

(ANOREXIANTS OR ANORECTICS)

Pharmacologic Management	Counseling Guidelines
Ingredients found in diet products: **Phenylpropanolamine (PPA) = Sympathomimetic Appetite suppressant via direct stimulation of satiety center of hypothalamus.** PPA 25 mg [Phenoxine] PPA 25 mg SR [Dexatrim Pre-Meal] PPA 37.5 mg [Prolamine] PPA 75 mg SR[MS Dexatrim, MS Dex-A-Diet, Acutrim 16 Hour, Acutrim Late Day, Acutrim II, MS] **Benzocaine** [Diet Ayds, Slim-Mint] **(local anesthetic) Æ Dysgeusia** [gums, candies, lozenges] **Dosing:** 6-15 mg before meals Maximum dose = 45 mg/day **Bulk Producers** (methylcellulose, carboxymethyl cellulose, agar, psyllium, and karaya gum)	1. Patients with diabetes, hypertension., heart disease, or thyroid disease should seek medical advice before taking products containing phenylpropanolamine 2. Allergic reactions may occur in some people taking benzocaine 3. Adequate fluid should always be used with bulk producers 4. Bulk products reduce hunger, but also create a laxative effect 5. Intestinal blockage can occur when one combines a prescribed drug for the stomach to slow intestinal movement, with a bulk-producing diet aid 6. PPA may interact with monoamine oxidase inhibitors (MAOIs) and tyramine-containing foods such as old cheese and stale meats to cause hypertensive crisis; indomethacin to cause psychotic reactions; and guanethidine (antagonism?). **Consult your pharmacist.**

Table 3b

WEIGHT AND DIET CONTROL PRODUCTS

(ANOREXIANTS OR ANORECTICS)

Pharmacologic Management	Counseling Guidelines

Non-Pharmacologic Management:
 	
1. Eat a low calorie balanced diet.
2. Use artificial sweeteners instead of sugar.
3. Exercise regularly.
4. Group therapy.
 	
Prescription Anorexiants/Anorectics:
 	
1. **Phentermine HCL** [Fastin, Adipex-P, Ionamin] 8 mg, 30 mg, 37.5 mg tablets (C-IV); 15 mg, 18.75 mg, 30 mg, 37.5 mg capsules (C-IV)
2. **Benzphetamine HCL** [Didrex] 25 mg, 50 mg tablets (C-III)
3. **Diethylpropion HCL** [Tenuate] 25 mg tablets, 75 mg SR tablets (C-IV)
4. **Fenfluramine HCL** [Pondimin] 20 mg tablets (C-IV) = Recalled
5. **Dexfenfluramine** [Redux] - Primary pulmonary hypertension!, often FATAL cardiovascular condition (Valvular Heart Disease). = Recalled
6. **Phendimetrazine tartrate** [Bontril PDM 35 mg tabs/caps (C-IV), Prelu-2, Rexigen Forte 105 mg caps SR (C-III)]
7. **Sibutramine HCL** [Meridia] = Impressive safety profile. No reported cases of primary pulmonary hypertension thus far.
 	
Indication: 8-12 weeks in combination with professionally supervised weight reduction program
	7. To obtain any of the prescription (Rx) anorexiants, a physician evaluation and prescription are required.
	
	8. Dexfenfluramine (Redux) has been associated with primary pulmonary hypertension. Consult your physician for routine evaluation if you are using this agent.
	
	9. The appetite stimulants, except the multivitamins, also require physician prescription before use.
	
	Appetite Stimulants available
	(E.g., in AIDS Wasting Syndrome) include:
	
	1. **Somatropin** [Serostim] 0.1mg/kg/d S.C. - Not FDA-Approved
	2. **Dronabinol** [Marinol (C-II)] 2.5 mg, 5 mg, 10 mg capsules 2 times/d.
	   - FDA-Approved
	3. **Megestrol Acetate** [Megace] 40 mg/ml suspension: 320-640 mg/d.
	   - Not FDA-Approved
	4. **Cyproheptadine HCL** [Periactin] 2 mg/5 ml syrup, 4 mg tablets (rx):4-20 mg/d. Initially 4 mg 3 times/d.
	5. **Multivitamins** (MVIs) - Not FDA-Approved
	6. **Corticosteroids;** e.g., Prednisone [Deltasone] 5mg/ml & 5mg/5ml oral solution, 5mg/5ml syrup, 1mg, 2.5mg, 5mg, 10mg, 20mg 50mg tablets: 5-60mg/d. - Not FDA-approved.
	7. **Oxymetholone** [Anadrol-50 (C-III)] 50mg tablets: 1-5mg/kg/d.
	   - Not FDA-Approved

24

INTERNAL ANALGESICS/ANTIPYRETICS

Products	Counseling Guidelines

Aspirin 80 mg or 325 mg
[Bayer, Empirin, Ecotrin=enteric-coated, Bufferin {325 mgASA+158 mg CaCO3+63 mg MgO+34 mg MgCO3}, Ascriptin, Ascriptin A/D {325 mg ASA+75 mg Mg(OH)2+ 75 mg Al(OH)3 & CaCO3}, Alka-Seltzer w/ASA {325 mg ASA+1.9 gm NaHCO3}]
Ibuprofen Suspension 100mg/5ml [Children's Motrin]
Ibuprofen 200 mg
[Motrin IB, Advil, Nuprin, Excedrin-IB*, Midol 200, Pamprin-IB, Medipren, Haltran]
Acetaminophen 325 mg or 500 mg
[Tylenol, Anacin-3, Panadol, Tempra, Dolanex]
Naproxen 200 mg (220 mg naproxen Na) [Aleve]
Ketoprofen [Orudis KT, Actron] 12.5 mg (75 mg/day).
Excedrin Migraine (ES) [acetaminophen + aspirin and caffeine] . . . . .
Mechanism of action: Inhibition of cyclo-oxygenase enzyme
 	
EXTERNAL ANALGESICS = COUNTERIRRITANTS:
Eucalyptus oil **(Flex-ALL 454, Flexerrall)** -cooling effect
Methyl salicylate **(Ben-Gay)** -reduces redness, irritation*
Turpentine oil **(Sloan's Liniment)** - reduces redness, irritation *
Menthol **(Ben-Gay)** - cooling effect
Camphor **(Vicks, VapoRub)** - cooling effect
Methyl Nicotinate **(Rid-A-Pain)** - vasodilator
Capsaicin creams 0.025%, 0.075% (**Zostrix, Zostrix-HP**)
- reduces irritation w/o redness.
- approx. equal to * in potency
(* Relatively more potent)
Dosage Forms: Liniments, gels, lotions, ointments
 	
12. Some external analgesic combinations available include
  a. Capsaicin + menthol [ArthiCare Ultra]
  b. Capsaicin + menthol + methyl salicylate [Pain Doctor]
	1. Do not exceed the maximum dosages on the product's label
	2. Adults should not take pain relievers for more than 10 days unless directed by a doctor
	3. Children and teenagers should limit use to five days for pain
	4. Because of the danger of Reye Syndrome, all children and young adults should not take aspirin for chicken pox, flu, or flu-like symptoms
	5. Those allergic to aspirin should not take any medicine containing aspirin-like ingredients such as carbaspirin calcium, choline salicylate, magnesium salicylate, and sodium salicylate. Signs of a reaction are itching, hives, runny nose, swelling of the throat, chest pains and fainting
	6. Pregnant women should not take aspirin especially in the last three months of pregnancy
	7. Avoid aspirin prior to surgery, unless directed otherwise by a doctor
	8. Enteric-coated aspirin products may reduce stomach upset
	9. Acetaminophen can be used in patients with a history of peptic ulcer disease
	10. Avoid the intermittent use of aspirin and oral anticoagulants (e.g., warfarin and heparin)
	11. Excedrin Migraine is the first OTC treatment for mild-to-moderate migraine headaches. It works by constricting blood vessels that are a source of migraine pain. Take 2 tablets at the first sign of a migraine, repeat every 6 hours as needed.

Table 4b

INTERNAL ANALGESICS/ANTIPYRETICS

Products	Counseling Guidelines
OTC URINARY TRACT INFECTION (UTI) PAIN RELIEF PRODUCTS (URINARY ANT-INFECTIVE ANALGESICS): Phenazopyridine HCL 95, 100, 200 mg **[Azo-Standard, Pyridium]:** OTC - 2 tablets after meals, 3 times daily for up to 2 days. Sulfamethoxazole 500 mg + Phenazopyridine HCL 100 mg **[Azo-Gantanol]:** Rx - 4 tablets initially, followed by 2 tablets q am and q pm for up to 2 days. Sulfisoxazole 500 mg+Phenazopyridine HCL 50 mg **[Azo-Gantrisin]:** Rx - 4 tablets initially, followed by 2 tablets 4 times daily for up to 2 days. Methenamine 40.8 mg+Phenyl salicylate 18.1 mg+Methylene blue 5.4 mg +Benzoic acid 4.5 mg+Atropine sulfate 0.03 mg+Hyoscyamine 0.03 mg **[Urised]:** Rx - 2 tablets 4 times daily. Oxytetracycline HCL 250 mg+Sulfamethizole 250 mg +Phenazopyridine HCL 50 mg **[Urobiotic-250]:** Rx - 1 capsule 4 times daily. - In refractory cases, 2 capsules 4 times daily.	12. Phenazopyridine (Pyridium)-containing medications may cause harmless and temporary discoloration of bodily excretions.the effectiveness of Pyridium alone as urinary analgesic is unknown since it is usually prescribed in combination with antibacterial agents.

Rx = Prescription (Medication can only be obtained by a written prescription from a physician).

26

ANTACIDS

Antacid Ingredient(s) .	Counseling Guidelines
Sodium Bicarbonate (NaHCO3) [Baking soda, Alka-Seltzer] **Calcium Carbonate (CaCO3)** [Titralac, Tums, Rolaids, Children's Mylanta] **Aluminum (AL)** [Amphogel, Alternagel] **Magnesium (Mg)** [Milk of Magnesia=MOM] **Magnesium + Aluminum combinations** [Maalox, Mylanta, Gelusil] **Other ingredients:** Sugar, **Simethicone** [Mylicon]-antiflatulent(gas) **Alginic acid(+NaHCO3),** **Bismuth Salts(Bismuth Subsalicylate) [Pepto-Bismol]**	1. Antacids for relief of indigestion symptoms should not be taken longer than 2 weeks 2. Antacids may cause diarrhea(Mg) or constipation (AL) 3. Magnesium containing antacids should be avoided in patients with chronic renal failure 4. Patients with diabetes should avoid antacids with sugar 5. Additional medications that the patient is taking should be identified to enable the pharmacist to monitor for drug interactions 6. Children's Mylanta (Calcium carbonate) is indicated for the relief of upset stomach in children 2 to 11 years of age. It is available in 400 mg bubble gum or fruit punch flavored liquid in 4 oz bottles or in chewable tablets in 24-count packages.

ANTACIDS

Antacid Ingredient	Counseling Guidelines
OTC H_2 - Antagonists = Low dose Cimetidine 200 mg [Tagamet HB,] Famotidine 10 mg [Pepcid AC, Mylanta AR ,] Ranitidine-75 mg [Zantac 75,] Ranitidine HCL 75 mg [Zantac 75 EFFERdose,] ** Nizatidine 75 mg [Axid AR,] Dosing: qd or bid prn X 2 weeks Rx Anti-Ulcer (H. pylori) Combinations: 1. Bismuth subsalicylate +metronidazole+tetracycline HCL [Helidac,] w/ an H_2-antagonist (e.g., Zantac) x 2 wks 2. Ranitidine bismuth citrate w/clarithromycin [Tritec,] x 4 wks, and 3. Omeprazole+clarithromycin x 4 wks	7. Significant Interactions w/Antacids: *Consult Pharmacist if you are taking any of the following medications:* Tetracyclines(decreased absorption), quinolone antibiotics (decreased absorption), digoxin/ digitoxin(decreased absorption), chlorpromazine(decreased absorption), quinidine(decreased absorption), indomethacin/ NSAIDS(decreased absorption), levodopa(variable), dexamethasone(decreased absorption), nitrofurantoin(decreased absorption), captopril(decreased absorption), H2-antagonists(decreased absorption), sucralfate(decreased dissolution/efficacy)*, theophylline(decreased absorption) **Note Mechanisms of Interaction:** A. decreased absorption via adsorption or chelation/complexation B. * Via increased pH C. Cimetidine+ Phenytoin or Warfarin or Theophylline result in increased levels of latter **Solution: Separate doses by 1-2 hours to avoid interaction with antacids.** ** Zantac 75 EFFERdose, is the first otc effervescent H2-antagonist to be approved by the FDA. The 75 mg efffervescent tablet is an alternative for people who have difficulty swallowing tablets.

ANTACIDS

COMPOSITION AND ACID NEUTRALIZING CAPACITY
OF SELECTED ANTACID PREPARATIONS
(Low Na+ Content)

Product	Dosage Forms	Aluminum (Mg/5ml)	Magnesium (Mg/5ml)	Calcium Carbonate (Mg/5ml)	Simethicone (Mg/5ml or Mg/Tablet or Water)	Acid Neutralizing Capacity (ANC)
Alternagel	Liquid	600				16
Aludrox	Suspension	307	103			12
Amphogel	Susp/Tabs/Tabs	320/300/600				10/8/16
Camalox	Susp/Tablet	225/225	200/200	250/250		18/18
Dicarbosil	Tablet			500		10
Di-Gel	Liquid	200	200		20	12
Gelusil	Liquid/Tablet	200/200	200/200		25/25	12/11
Gelusil-II	Susp/Tablet	400/400	400/400		30/30	24/21
Maalox	Susp/Tablet	225/200	200/200			13/10
Maalox-ES	Tablet	400	400			23
Maalox Plus	Tablet	200	200		25	11
Maalox Plus-ES	Liquid	500	450		40	29
Maalox-TC	Liquid/Tablet	600/600	300/300			27/28
Milk of Magnesia	Susp/Tablet		390/325			14/11
Mylanta	Susp/Tablet	200/200	200/200		20/20	13
Mylanta-II	Susp/Tablet	400/400	400/400		40/40	25/23
Riopan(Magaldrate)	Susp/Tablet	540/480				15/14
Riopan-ES	Suspension	1080				30
Riopan Plus	Susp/Tablet	540/480			20/20	15/14
Riopan Plus 2	Susp/Tablet	1080/1080			30/30	30/30
Tempo	Tablet	133	81	414	20	14
Titralac	Tablet			420		8
Titralac Plus	Liquid			500	20	11
Tums	Tablet			500		10
Tums-ES	Liquid			1000		20
Tums E-X	Tablet			750		15
Wingel	Susp/Tablet	180/180	160/160			12/12

Table 6a

ANTIDIARRHEALS

Pharmacologic Management	Counseling Guidelines
Adsorbents: **Attapulgite** [Kaopectate 600 mg, Children's Kaopectate 300 mg, Kaopectate-MS 750 mg, Donnagel 600 mg, Diasorb 750 mg, parepectolin 600 mg, Rheaban-MS 750 mg, K-Pek 600 mg/15 ml, K-C, Kaodene Non-Narcotic] chewable tablets, caplets, liquid 　　Kaolin-Pectin [Kapectolin] 　　Activated charcoal 　　Aluminum hydroxide 　　Magnesium trisilicate **Bismuth Salts are Antimicrobials** **Bismuth Subsalicylate (BSS)** [Pepto-Bismol 262 mg/15 ml, Pink Bismuth 262 mg/15 ml, Bismatrol, Bismatrol Extra Strength 524 mg/15 ml, Pepto-Bismol Maximum Strength 524 mg/15 ml] 262 mg (Total Salicylates 99-102 mg) caplets, liquid, chewable tablets Dose: 2 tablets or 30 ml q1/2-1h prn, up to 8 doses in 24 hours **Opioid-like Agents decrease peristalsis** **Loperamide [Imodium, Imodium AD,** Kaopectate II Caplets, Maalox Anti-Diarrheal Caplets, Pepto Diarrhea Control] 2 mg tablets, capsules, and liquid 1 mg/5 ml: Dose: 4 mg followed by 2 mg after each unformed stool. Do not exceed 16 mg/day. **Anticholinergics** **(Rx) decrease peristalsis** 　Belladonna alkalloids (Rx), Atropine (Rx) 　Hyoscyamine (Rx), Scopolamine (Rx) **Miscellaneous Agents:** 　Polycarbophil=Synthetic resin adsorbent 　**Forms:** 500 mg chewable tablets 　**Dose:** 4-6 gm/day in divided doses.	1. Avoid in children under 3 years of age 2. Avoid in patients over 60 years of age who have multiple conditions 3. Avoid in patients with a history of chronic illness such as asthma, peptic ulcer disease, diabetes, or heart disease 4. Avoid in pregnant patients 5. Do not use for more than 2 days or in the presence of high fever, bloody stools, or abdominal tenderness 6. Patients who are sensitive to aspirin should not use Pepto-Bismol 7. Drink plenty of fluids. 8. Follow dosing instructions on the packet. 9. A darkened coating on the tongue may occur from Bismuth salts. Darkening of the stool is also possible. Both conditions are harmless and temporary.

ANTIDIARRHEALS

Pharmacologic and Nonpharmacologic Management	

Non-Pharmacologic Management:
 	
1. Drink small amount of flat cola or ginger ale
2. Drink Gatorade or Pedialyte
3. Avoid milk for 10 days
 	
Note: PRESCRIPTION GI ANTICHOLINERGIC COMBINATIONS
 	
Belladonna Extract 15 mg+Butabarbital 15 mg Na+Alcohol 7%, Sucrose, Saccharin **[Butibel Elixir]:** 20-40 ml daily.
 	
Atropine sulfate 0.195 mg+Phenobarbital 16 mg+Alcohol 20% **[Atrocol Elixir]:** 15-40 ml daily.
 	
Hyoscyamine sulfate 0.125 mg+Phenobarbital 15 mg+Alcohol 5% **[Levsin PB Drops]:** 6-12 ml daily.
 	
Atropine sulfate 0.0194 mg+Scopolamine Hbr 0.0065 mg +Hyoscyamine sulfate 0.1037 mg+Phenobarbital 16.2 mg **[Donnatal]:** 1-2 capsules or tablets by mouth 3-4 times daily.
   - Elixir (per 5 ml) - contains alcohol 23%
    5-10 ml by mouth 3-4 times daily.
 	
Atropine sulfate 0.0582 mg+Scopolamine Hbr 0.0195 mg +Hyoscyamine sulfate 0.3111 mg+Phenobarbital 48.6 mg **[Donnatal Extentabs]** - SR tablets: 1 tablet by mouth q8-12h.
 	
DiphenoxylateHCL 2.5 mg+Atropine sulfate 0.025 mg+Alcohol 15% **[Lomotil, Lonox=Rx & C-V]** - tablets, liquid/ 5 ml.
10 ml po 4 times daily until control of diarrhea is achieved.
2 tablets po 4 times daily until control of diarrhea is achieved
	10. Anticholinergic side effects may result from the use of the anticholinergic agents which may manifest as dry mouth, urinary retention, blurred vision and constipation. Consult with your pharmacist if you experience any of these symptoms.

Table 7a

LAXATIVES

Pharmacologic and Non-Pharmacologic Management	Counseling Guidelines
Bulk-producing Laxatives: **1 tbsp (19 g)/8 oz cold water, 1-3 times/d** Methylcellulose [Citrucel] Cellulose [Unifiber] Psyllium [Metamucil, Fiberall Natural/Orange Flavor, Hydrocil Instant, Konsyl, Reguloid] Polycarbophil[Mitrolan, Fiberall, Fiber-Con, Fiber-Lax, Equalactin] **Stool Softeners or Emollients:** Docusate Sodium(DSS)[Colace] 50 mg, 100mg, 240 mg, 250 mg capsules: 50-500 mg/d DSS+Casanthranol[Peri-Colace]100mg capsules: 1-2 cap/d Docusate Calcium[Surfak] 50mg, 240mg: 1 capsule/d Docusate Potassium [Dialose, Kasof] 100 mg tablets, 240 mg capsules: 100-300 mg/d **Lubricants:** Mineral Oil[Kondremul] 5-45 ml/d **Saline Laxatives:** Magnesium sulfate[Epsom salts]10-15g/glass H2O Magnesium citrate[Mag Citrate] 240 ml prn **Irritant or Stimulant Laxatives:** Bisacodyl[Dulcolax]5 mg EC: 10-15 mg/d Phenolphthalein[Ex-Lax*, Feen-A-Mint] 60-194 mg/d Senna[Senokot, Senexon, Senolax] 187 mg, 2-8 tablets/d Aloe cascara sagrada (Nature's Remedy) 325 mg /d **Enemas for Rectal Administration** Phosphate compounds [Fleet Enema] 118 ml **Osmotic Laxatives:** Milk of magnesia[Phillips MOM]30-60 ml/d Lactulose [Chronulac,Cephulac] 15-30 ml/d **Laxative Combinations: 1-2 qhs with glass of H$_2$O** DSS+Senna[Senokot-S 50/187, Gentlax-S 50/8.6] DSS+Phenolphthalein **[Doxidan 60/65, Correctol 100/65, Femilax 100/65]**	1. Laxatives are not designed for long-term use. 2. Saline laxative should not be used daily and should not be given to children under 6 years of age. 3. Mineral oil should not be given to children under 6 years of age or in conjunction with emollient laxatives; they should not be used during pregnancy and should be avoided in patients taking anticoagulants and elderly (leakage in elderly). 4. Laxatives should not be used in the presence of abdominal pain, nausea, vomiting, or cramping. 5. Laxatives containing cascara sagrada, casanthranol, senna (Anthraquinones) or phenolphthalein may discolor urine. 6. Avoid docusate sodium in congestive heart failure (CHF) and/or hypertension (HTN). Use docusate calcium instead. 7. Consult your pharmacist for directions for use of enemas. They are formulated for RECTAL administration. 8. Suppositories should be inserted RECTALLY. Remove the aluminum foil prior to insertion. 9. Keep all suppositories refrigerated NOT frozen. 10. Animal studies show that phenolphthalein may be associated with cancer. Novartis is temporarily removing its laxative, Ex-Lax (phenolphthalein), from the market. 11. Metamucil also functions as a stool softener.

32

Table 7b

LAXATIVES

Pharmacologic and Non-Pharmacologic Management	Counseling Guidelines
Miscellaneous Products: Glycerin suppositories [Sani-Supp, Fleet Babylax 4 ml per applicator] Castor oil [Purge, Emulsoil] 15-60 ml/d **Non-Pharmacologic Management:** 1. Adequate fiber in diet. 2. Regular, mild exercise. 3. Adequate fluid intake. 4. Relaxation to reduce emotional stress and its effect on defecation. Note: MECHANISMS OF ACTION OF LAXATIVES: 1. **Bulk-Producers:** Natural or synthetic polysaccharide derivatives that adsorb water to soften stool and increase bulk, which stimulates peristalsis. 2. **Stool Softeners or Emollients:** Act as surfactants by allowing absorption of water into the stool, which makes the softened stool easier to pass. 3. **Saline and Osmotic Laxatives:** Work by creating an osmotic gradient to pull water into the small and large intestine. This increased volume results in distention of the intestinal lumen resulting in increased peristalsis and bowel motility. 4. **Irritant or Stimulant Laxatives:** Work in the small and large intestine to stimulate bowel motility and increase the secretion of fluids into the bowel.	Constant and adequate non-pharmacologic approaches may help avoid the use of drug products.

Table 8

HEMORRHOIDALS

Pharmacologic Management	Counseling Guidelines
Local Anesthetics:→ **relieve pain, burning, itching and irritation** Benzocaine [Americaine oint./suppos] Pramoxine HCL [Anusol H oint./suppos] **Vasoconstrictors:**→ **sympathomimetics/reduce swelling and congestion of anorectal tissue(Rx).** Ephedrine Epinephrine Phenylephrine Pazo & Wyanoids hemorrhoidal suppos **Protectants:** Lanolin Petrolatum (probably the best) Cocoa butter Calamine Mineral oil Shark liver oil [Preparation H oint./suppos] **Astringent:**→ **shrink swollen tissue** Hamarnelis Water[Witchhazel] in Tuck pads Preparation H Cleansing Pads **Corticosteroids: Rx = (See Pharmacist)** → reduce swelling & inflammation 2.5% Hydrocortisone cream[Anusol-HC] 25 mg Hydrocortisone acetate [Anucort-HC, Anusol-HC, Hemril-HC Uniserts, Hemor rhoidal-HC]	1. For maximum effect, non-prescription anorectal products should be after bowel movements rather than before. 2. If seepage, bleeding, and/or protrusion occurs, contact a physician. 3. Products designed for external use only should not be inserted into the rectum. 4. If insertion of a product in the rectum causes pain, stop the product and contact a physician. 5. Wash the anorectal area with warm water before applying any product. 6. If symptoms do not improve after 7 days, contact a physician. 7. Avoid eating spicy foods. Eat a diet high in fiber and fluid. 8. Patients with heart disease, diabetes, and hypertension should avoid products containing a vasoconstrictor. 9. Remove aluminum foil prior to rectal insertion of suppositories. 10. Keep all suppositories refrigerated NOT frozen.

Table 9

ANTIEMETICS AND EMETICS

Pharmacologic Products	Use or Indication and Counseling Guidelines

ANTIEMETICS
 	
Antihistamines: → **prevent nausea & vomiting** **sensations**
    Cyclizine HCL 50mg[Marezine]
    Meclizine HCL 25mg [Antivert, Bonine, Dizmiss]
    Dimenhydrinate 12.5mg, 50mg
    (diphenhydramine+chlorotheophylline 1:1)
                [Dramamine, Marmine, Calm-X]
 	
Phosphorated carbohydrate
    (levulose+dextrose+phosphoric acid mixture)
    [Emetrol]
 	
EMETICS
    Syrup of **ipecac** → **induce nausea & vomiting**
	Antihistamines are used for prevention of motion sickness
	
	Emetrol is used for nausea and vomiting associated with upset stomach caused by intestinal flu.
	
	Ipecac is used to induce vomiting in cases of oral poisoning
	
	Note:
	
	1. Abuse potential by Bulimics associated with Ipecac
	
	2. Ipecac contains toxic alkaloids (emetine and cephaeline)

35

Table 10a

COUGH/COLD/ALLERGY PRODUCTS

Decongestants	Antihistamines	Antitussives	Expectorants
Oral decongestants Phenylephrine HCL 10, 20, 40 mg [Deconsal, Endal, Sinupan] Phenylpropanolamine 25, 50, 75 mg [Propagest] Pseudoephedrine 30, 60, 120 mg [Sudafed, Efidac, Afrin] *Short-acting topical decongestants* Ephedrine sulfate 0.1% [Vicks Vatronol] Phenylephrine HCL 0.125-1% [Neo-Synephrine] *Long-acting deconges-tants* Oxymetazoline HCL 0.025, 0.05% [Allerest, Duration] Xylometazoline HCL 0.05, 0.1% [Otrivin] *Product information* May cause sleeplessness. May increase blood pressure or cause arrhythmias. Contraindicated in heart disease, HTN, diabetes, hyperthyroidism, patients taking MAO inhibitors, tyramine containing foods.	Alkylamines: Brompheniramine maleate [Dimetane] 8, 12 mg Chlorpheniramine maleate [Chlor-Trimeton, Tranquil] 4, 8, 12 mg Ethanolamines: Diphenhydramine HCL [Benadryl] 25, 50 mg Miscellaneous: Triprolidine HCL [Actidil] 1.25 mg/5 ml, 2.5 mg Clemastine Fumerate [Tavist-1] 1.34, 2.68 mg Azelastine [Astelin] Nasal Spray - **Rx only** (bitter taste, somnolence, wt. gain, myalgia, headache nasal burning, **no interaction with erythromycin**) *Product Information* May cause drowsiness. May produce a drying effect. May cause dry mouth, blurred vision, urinary retention. Note: **For dry mouth, Saliva Substitutes or Artificial Saliva such as Saliva Substitute, Optimoist, Moi-Stir, Moi-Stir Swab-Sticks, Entertainer's Secret, Salivart, Mouth Kote Solutions, and Salix Lozenges may be helpful.**	Codeine sulfate 15, 30, 60 mg Dextromethorphan [St. Joseph Cough Suppressant] 2.5, 3.5, 7.5 mg Diphenhydramine HCL [Benadryl, Diphen Cough] 25, 50 mg *Product Information* Codeine may cause drowsiness, sedation nausea, and constipation. Codeine is contraindicated in patients with increased intracranial pressure and should be used cautiously in COPD, head injuries, hepatic or renal diseases, or a history of drug or alcohol abuse. Dextromethorphan may cause drowsiness and GI distress. Note: **Formulations may also contain analgesics such as aspirin, acetaminophen, and non-steroidal anti-inflammatory drugs (NSAIDs) and excipients such as caffeine, sucrose, dextrose, sugar, and sorbitol. Some of these excipients could be clinically important in certain patients (e.g., sorbitol rather than sucrose or sugar or dextrose preferred for diabetics).**	Guaifenesin 100, 200 mg, 300 mg, 600 mg [Robitussin, Guaituss, Hytuss, Naldecon, Organidin, Humibid] **Robitussin A-C (C-V), Robitussin-CF, Robitussin-DM ... etc** (Consult Package and/or Pharmacist) → with large doses, may cause nausea or vomiting Terpin hydrate **Elixir** 85 mg/5 ml **Water = Best expectorant** *Guidelines on when to consult a physician for "cold" symptoms* Cough lasting beyond 2 weeks. Discolored or bloody mucus from respiratory passages. Pain or tenderness around eyes: severe headache. Pain or wheezing on breathing: shortness of breath. Fever > 100.5 F beyond two days, or sore throat beyond three days. White patches on back of throat or tonsils: red throat. Chronic, debilitating fatigue. Cold symptoms become more severe than usual, or localized in throat, stomach or lungs. Vomiting occurs, and persists beyond a day.

Table 10b

COUGH/COLD/ALLERGY PRODUCTS

Examples of Common Combination Products	Examples of Common Combination Products
Consult Pharmacist or Medication Label for Directions and precautionary measures.	
Dristan Cold Multi-Symptom [phenylephrine 5 mg +chlorpheniramine 2 mg+APAP 325 mg +caffeine]	**Deconamine** [pseudoephedrine 30 mg+chlorpheniramine 2 mg]
Drixoral Cold & Flu [pseudoephedrine 60 mg +dexbrompheniramine 3 mg+APAP 500 mg]	**Entex LA** [PPA 75 mg+guaifenesin 400 mg]
Actifed [pseudoephedrine 60 mg+triprolidine 2.5 mg]	**Hycotuss Expectorant (C-III)** [hydrocodone bitartrate 5 mg+guaifenesin 100 mg+alcohol 10%]
Actifed Plus [pseudoephedrine 30 mg+triprolidine 1.25 mg +APAP 500 mg]	**Naldecon-CX (C-V)** [codeine 10 mg+PPA 12.5 mg +guaifenesin 200 mg]
Actifed w/Codeine(C-V) [Actifed Plus+codeine 10 mg +alcohol 4.3%]	**Novahistine DMX** [dextromethorphan 10 mg +pseudoephedrine 30 mg+guaifenesin 100 mg+alcohol 10%]
Dimetapp Allergy Sinus [PPA 12.5 mg+brompheniramine 2 mg]	**Ornade** [PPA 75 mg+chlorpheniramine 12 mg] - SR capsules
Tavist-D [PPA 75 mg+clemastine fumarate 1.34 mg]	**Rondec-DM** [pseudoephedrine 60 mg+carbinoxamine maleate 4 mg+dextromethorphan 15 mg]
Allerest Pain Formula [pseudoephedrine 30 mg +chlorpheniramine 2 mg+APAP 500 mg]	**Sinutab Sinus Allergy Medication, Maximum Strength** [pseudoephedrine 30 mg+chlorpheniramine 2 mg+APAP 500 mg]
Ambenyl (C-V) [codeine 10 mg+bromodiphenhydramine 12.5 mg+alcohol 5%]	**Triaminicol Multisymptom Cold Tablets** [PPA 12.5 mg +chlorpheniramine 2 mg+dextromethorphan 10 mg]
Benadryl Allergy Decongestant [pseudoephedrine 60 mg +diphenhydramine 25 mg]	**Tussionex (C-III)** [chlorpheniramine polistirex 8 mg+hydrocodone polistirex 10 mg] - SR Suspension (per 5 ml)
Benylin Multisymptom [dextromethorphan 5 mg +guaifenesin 100 mg+pseudoephedrine 15 mg]	**Tussi-Organidin DM NR** [dextromethorphan 10 mg+guaifenesin 100 mg]
Cheracol D [dextromethorphan 10 mg+guaifenesin 100 mg +alcohol 4.75%]	**Nyquil Adult Nighttime Cold Flu Medicine** [doxylamine succinate, 12.5mg / 30 mL acetaminophen, 1000 mg/30mL, dextromethorphan HBr 30mg/30mL, alcohol, 25%]
Comtrex [dextromethorphan 15 mg+pseudoephedrine 30 mg +chlorpheniramine 2 mg+APAP 500 mg]	
Coricidin "D" [PPA 12.5 mg+chlorpheniramine 2 mg +APAP 325 mg]	

COUGH/COLD/ALLERGY PRODUCTS

Non-Sedating Antihistamines & Miscellaneous Agents	Counseling Guidelines

Second Generation Antihistamines-Rx
 	
Seldane [Terfenadine 60 mg] = recalled!
Seldane-D [Terfenadine 60mg +Pseudoephedrine 120mg]
  = recalled!
Allegra [Fexofenadine 60 mg]
Allegra-D [Fexofenadine+Pseudoephedrine]
  = FDA-approved
Hismanal [Astemizole 10mg]
Optimine [Azatadine1mg]
Claritin [Loratadine10mg]
Claritin-D [Loratadine 5mg+Pseudoephedrine 120mg] 12-hour SR
Claritin-D [Loratadine 10mg+Pseudoephedrine 240mg] 24-hour SR
Zyrtec [Cetirizine 5, 10 mg]
 	
Miscellaneous Products:
 	
Nasalcrom [Cromolyn sodium nasal solution]
Indication: Allergic rhinitis.
Dose: 1 spray in each nostril 3-4 times daily at regular intervals for 2-4 weeks.
Vancenase AQ [Beclomethasone nasal spray 84 mcg]
Indication: Allergic and non-allergic rhinitis.
Dose: 1 inhalation (42 mcg) in each nostril 2-4 times daily.
Atrovent [Intranasal Ipratropium Bromide 84 mcg]
  or
Intranasal Atropine
Indication: Rhinorrhea and sneezing associated with common colds?
Dose: 1 spray per nostril 3-4 times daily.
	Note the following potentially fatal Adverse Drug Reactions (ADRs) or Interactions:
	
	Interaction between terfenadine (Seldane) & ketoconazole, erythromycin, hepatic dysfunction resulting in arrhythmias, QT Interval prolongation, death.
	
	Similar interactions may occur between astemizole (Hismanal) and erythromycin. Loratadine has not been shown to interact with either macrolides or -azole antifungals; hence is a safe alternative to use in combination.
	
	Other -azole antifungal agents such as fluconazole and itraconazole and the newer macrolides such as clarithromycin and azithromycin may also be incompatible with terfenadine (Seldane) and astemizole (Hismanal). Caution must be exercised whenever these two categories of medications are prescribed for concurrent use.
	
	In fact, concurrent use should be discouraged. Inform your pharmacist of all the medications you are currently taking.

VITAMINS AND MINERALS

Multivitamin Indicators	Patient Information
1. **Iatrogenic situations:** oral contraceptive and estrogen users, patients on prolonged broad-spectrum antibiotics, patients receiving isoniazid, or patients on prolonged total parenteral nutrition 2. **Inadequate dietary intake conditions:** alcoholics, the impoverished, the aged, or patients on severe calorie-restricted diet of fad diets 3. **Increased metabolic requirements:** pregnant or lactating women, infants, or patients with severe injury, trauma, major surgery, or severe infections 4. **Poor absorption:** the aged, or patients with such conditions as prolonged diarrhea, severe GI disorders and malignancy, surgical removal of sections of the GI tract, celiac disease, obstructive jaundice, or cystic fibrosis	1. Read the labels on all vitamin or vitamin and mineral preparations before you take them. Compare the contents and the amounts of vitamins and minerals with the RDAs. 2. Take vitamins or vitamin and mineral supplements with meals. Iron supplements may cause less stomach upset/constipation if taken with meals. 3. Do not take high doses of vitamins or minerals; high doses may be dangerous. It is best not to exceed the RDA. Follow label directions. 4. Do not self-medicate for a vitamin deficiency. If you believe that you are vitamin deficient, consult your physician or pharmacist 5. For proper nutrition, eat foods from all basic food groups (meats, fruits and vegetable, dairy products, and grains). Vitamin supplements are not a substitute for a well-balanced diet. 6. Liquid vitamin and mineral supplements may be mixed with food (fruit juice, milk, baby formula, or cereal). 7. Iron supplements or vitamins with iron may turn stool black. 8. Niacin- containing products may cause a flushing sensation. Aspirin will prevent flushing.

Table 11b

VITAMINS AND MINERALS

VITAMIN	NAME	USE or INDICATION
Vitamin A (Beta-Carotene)	Retinol 100,000 IU cream, Retinol-A 300,000 IU cream, Aquasol A 5,000 IU/0.1 ml Drops, Palmitate-A 5000 5,000 IU tablets, Vitamin A 10,000 IU capsules	Retinal function, Bone growth
Vitamin B1	Thiamine Hcl 50, 100, 250, 500 mg tablets, Thiamilate 20 mg Enteric-Coated (EC) tablets	Carbohydrate metabolism
Vitamin B2	Riboflavin 25, 50, 100 mg tablets	Tissue respiration
Vitamin B3	Niacin; Nicotinic Acid 25, 50, 100, 250, 500 mg tablets, Slo-Niacin 250, 500, 750 mg SR tablets, Nicotinic Acid (Niacin) 125, 250 mg SR capsules, Nicobid Tempules 125, 250, 500 mg SR capsules, Niac 300 mg SR capsules, Nicotinic Acid (Niacin) 400, 500 mg SR capsules, Nia-Bid, Niacels, Nico-400 400mg SR capsules, Nicotinex 50 mg/5 ml **Elixir**	Lipid metabolism
Vitamin B6	Pyridoxine Hcl 25, 50, 100 mg tablets, Nestrex 25 mg tablets, Vitamin B6 100 mg SR tablets	Amino acid metabolism, Prevention or treatment of peripheral neuropathy secondary to isoniazid use
Vitamin B9	Folic acid (Folate) 0.4, 0.8 mg tablets, Folic acid (Folate) 1 mg tablets = Rx only	Red blood cell formation, Megaloblastic anemia
Vitamin B12	Cyanocobalamin 25, 50, 100, 250 mcg tablets, Ener-B 400 mcg/unit **Nasal gel** **Dose: 1 tablet/d qhs with full glass of water**	Red blood cell formation, Megaloblastic anemia

VITAMINS AND MINERALS

VITAMIN	NAME	USE OR INDICATION
Vitamin C	Ascorbic Acid 25, 50, 100, 250, 500, 1000 mg tablets, Ascorbic Acid 100, 250, 500, tablets, Chewable, Ascorbic Acid Caplets 500, 1000, 1500 mg SR tablets, Ascorbic Acid, Ascorbicap, Cebid Timecelles, Cetane, Cevi-Bid, 500 mg SR capsules, N'ice Vitamin C Drops 60 mg Lozenges, Vita-C, 4 gm/5 ml crystals, Dull-C, 4 gm /5 ml powder, Ce-Vi-Sol 35 mg/0.6 ml Liquid, Cecon 100 mg/ml solution, Ascorbic Acid 500 mg syrup, Sodium Ascorbate 585 mg tablets = 500 mg ascorbic acid, Sodium Ascorbate 1020 mg crystals=900 mg ascorbic acid, Calcium Ascorbate 610 mg tablets=500 mg ascorbic acid, Calcium Ascorbate 1 gm Powder=826 mg ascorbic acid, **Ascorbic Acid Combinations:** Chewable C tablets (100, 250, 300, 500 mg Vit. C as Na ascorbate+ascorbic acid), Vicks Vitamin C Drops Lozenges (60 mg Vit. C as Na ascorbate+ascorbic acid)	Collagen formation, Tissue repair

Table 11d

VITAMINS AND MINERALS

VITAMIN	NAME	USE OR INDICATION
Vitamin D2	Ergocalciferol, Calciferol Drops 8,000 IU/ml Drisdol Drops 8,000 IU/ml	Absorption + utilization of calcium and phosphate
Vitamin D3	Cholecalciferol, Delta-D 400 IU D3 tablets, Vitamin D3 1000 IU D3 tablets	Absorption + utilization of calcium and phosphate
Vitamin E	Tocopherol, Aquasol E 73.5 mg capsules, E-200 I.U. Softgels 147 mg capsules, E-Vitamin Succinate 165 mg capsules, Amino-Opti-E 165 mg capsules, Aquasol E 400 IU capsules, E-400 I.U. capsules in a Water Soluble Base, E-Vitamin Succinate 330 mg capsules, Vita-Plus E Softgels 400 IU capsules, E-Complex-600 IU capsules, E-1000 I.U. Softgels 1000 IU capsules, Aquasol E 50 mg/ml Drops	Antioxidant
Vitamin K1	Phytonadione 2 mg/ml injection (aqueous colloidal solution) - Rx	Blood clotting
Vitamin K3	Menadione	Blood clotting

VITAMINS AND MINERALS

MINERALS AND TRACE ELEMENTS	NAME	USE OR INDICATION
Calcium	**Calcium Carbonate, 40% Calcium:** Calcium carbonate 650 mg tablets (260 mg Ca), Calciday 667 667 mg tablets (266.8 mg Ca), Calcium carbonate, Os-Cal 500, Oyst-Cal 500, Oystercal 500, **Oyster Shell Calcium-500:** 1.25 gm (500 mg Ca), Calcium 600, Cal-Plus, Caltrate 600, Gencalc 600, Nephro-Calci: 1.5 gm (600 mg Ca), Caltrate, Jr. 750 mg (300 mg Ca) tablets, chewable, Calci-Chew, Os-Cal 500, Oysco 500: 1.25 gm (500 mg Ca) tablets, chewable, Calci-Mix 1250 mg (500 mg Ca) powder capsules, Calcium carbonate 1.25 gm (500 mg Ca)/5 ml oral suspension, Cal Carb-HD 6.5 gm (2400 mg Ca) per packet powder, Florical 364 mg (145.6 mg Ca)+8.3 mg sodium fluoride capsules & tablets: 1 capsule or tablet/day **Calcium Gluconate, 9% Calcium:** Calcium gluconate 500 mg (45 mg Ca) tablets, Calcium gluconate 650 mg (58.5 mg Ca) tablets, Calcium gluconate 975 mg (87.75 mg Ca) tablets, Calcium gluconate 1 gm (90 mg Ca) tablets Calcium Glubionate, 6.5% Calcium Neo-Calglucon 1.8 gm (115 mg Ca) syrup **Calcium Lactate, 13% Calcium:** Calcium lactate 325 mg (42.25 mg Ca) tablets, Calcium lactate 650 mg (84.5 mg Ca) tablets, Tricalcium phosphate (Ca Phosphate), 39% Ca Posture 1565.2 mg (600 mg Ca) **Calcium Citrate, 21% Calcium:** Citracal 950 mg (200 mg Ca) tablets, Citracal Liquitab 2376 mg (500 mg Ca) tablets, effervescent **Calcium Acetate, 25% Calcium:** Phos-Ex 62.5 Mini-Tabs 250 mg (62.5 mg Ca), Phos-Ex 167 668 mg (167 mg Ca), Phos-Ex 250 1000 mg (250 mg Ca); Phos-Ex 125 500 mg (125 mg Ca) capsules: 500 mg-2 gm 2-4 times/day	Bones and teeth growth, blood clotting and prevention of osteoporosis and osteomalacia. Note: 1. Taking calcium with food increases absorption, particularly calcium carbonate. Calcium carbonate absorption is impaired in patients with achlorhydria. Whether H-2-receptor antagonists or proton pump inhibitors have a similar effect has not been determined 2. Calcium supplements are usually well tolerated in doses up to 1,500 mg per day. GI effects such as constipation, intestinal bloating and excess gas have been reported, particularly with calcium carbonate. 3. Switching preparations or increasing fluid intake may relieve the problem. Calcium carbonate is relatively inexpensive, has a large amount of elemental calcium per tablet and is generally well tolerated but may cause more GI adverse effects than calcium citrate or calcium phosphate.

Table 11f

VITAMINS AND MINERALS

MINERALS AND TRACE ELEMENTS	NAME	USE OR INDICATION
Chromium	Chromium chloride Chromium Picolinate 200 mcg Chromium tablets: 10-15 mcg/day	Proper glucose utilization to produce energy ("glucose tolerance factor") and Fat (cholesterol) metabolism.
Copper	Copper, Cupric sulfate: 0.5-1.5 mg/day	Enzyme co-factor, involved in the storage and release of the iron needed to form hemoglobin for red blood cells.
Chlorine	Sodium chloride, Potassium chloride	Essential electrolyte.
Fluoride	Sodium fluoride: (See directions accompanying the product)	Protection against dental caries.
Iodine	Potassium iodide: 1-2 mcg/kg/day (75-150 mcg/day)	Thyroid gland (goiter) function, incorporated in thyroxin and tri-iodothyronine hormones for maintaining the body metabolic rate.

Table 11g

VITAMINS AND MINERALS

MINERALS AND TRACE ELEMENTS	NAME	USE OR INDICATION
Iron	**Ferrous sulfate (natural), 20% elemental iron (Fe)** Mol-iron 195 mg (39 mg Fe) tablets, Feratab 300 mg (60 mg Fe) tablets, Ferrous sulfate 324 mg (65 mg Fe) tablets, Ferrous sulfate, Ferrospace 250 mg (50 mg Fe) capsules, Fero-Gradumet Filmtab 525 mg (105 mg Fe) SR tablets, Fer-In-Sol 90 mg (18 mg Fe) syrup, Ferrous sulfate, Feosol 220 mg (44 mg Fe) elixir, Ferrous sulfate, Fer-In-Sol 75 mg (15 mg Fe) drops Fer-Iron 125 mg (25 mg Fe) per ml drops, **Ferrous Sulfate Exsiccated (Dried):** Fer-In-Sol 190 mg (60 mg Fe) capsules, Feosol 200 mg (65 mg Fe) tablets, Feosol 159 mg (50 mg Fe) SR capsules, Ferrous sulfate, Ferralyn Lanacaps, Ferra-TD 250 mg (50 mg Fe) capsules, Slow FE 160 mg (50 mg Fe) SR tablets, **Ferrous gluconate, 11.6% elemental Fe:** Ferrous gluconate 300 mg (34 mg Fe) tablets, Fergon, Ferralet 320 mg (37 mg Fe) tablets, Ferrous gluconate 325 mg (38 mg Fe) SR tablets, Ferralet Slow Release 320 mg (37 mg Fe) SR tablets, Simron 86 mg (10 mg Fe) capsules, soft gelatin, Fergon 300 mg (34 mg Fe) **elixir,**	Used in hemoglobin to carry oxygen, enzyme co-factor, prevention of iron deficiency anemia. **Note:** 1. May cause constipation and black, tarry stools. 2. Vitamin C helps the body use iron more effectively by enhancing absorption of iron. 3. Iron will decrease absorption of tetracycline and allopurinol. 4. Docusate sodium may alleviate or prevent the constipation.

Table 11h

VITAMINS AND MINERALS

MINERALS AND TRACE ELEMENTS	NAME	USE OR INDICATION
Iron (continued)	**Ferrous fumarate, 33% elemental Fe**: Femiron 63 mg (20 mg Fe) tablets, Fumerin 195 mg (64 mg Fe) tablets, Fumasorb, Ircon 200 mg (66 mg Fe) tablets, Hemocyte 324 mg (106 mg Fe) tablets, Ferrous fumarate 325 mg (106 mg Fe) tablets, Nephro-Fer 350 mg (115 mg Fe) tablets, Feostat 100 mg (33 mg Fe) tablets, chewable, Span-FF 325 mg (106 mg Fe) SR capsules, Feostat 100 mg (33 mg Fe) per 5 ml suspension, Feostat 45 mg (15 mg Fe) per 0.6 ml drops, **Polysaccharide-Iron Complex**: Niferex 50 mg Fe tablets, Hytinic, Niferex-150, Nu-Iron 150 mg Fe capsules, Niferex, Nu-Iron 100 mg Fe per 5 ml elixir **Modified Iron Products**: Fermalox 200 mg Fe sulfate tablets (40 mg Fe)+100 mg $Mg(OH)_2$+100 mg $Al(OH)_3$ Ferocyl, Ferr-Sequels 150 mg Fe fumarate (50 mg Fe)+100 mg docusate sodium (DSS) SR tablets, Ferro-Docusate T.R.. Ferro Dok TR, Ferro-DSS S.R. 150 mg Fe fumarate (50 mg Fe)+100 mg DSS SR capsules, **Iron With Vitamin C**: Mol-Iron with Vitamin C, Ferancee-HP, Vitron-C-Plus, tablets; Niferex with Vitamin C, Vitron-C, Ferancee, tablets, chewable **Capsules and Tablets, Timed Release (SR)**: Irospan, Fe-O.D., Fero-Grad-500 Filmtabs, Hemaspan 10-30 mg/day (RDA) **[Iron Dextran (InFeD) = Rx]**	

VITAMINS AND MINERALS

MINERALS AND TRACE ELEMENTS	NAME	USE OR INDICATION
Magnesium	Magnesium sulfate (Epsom salts), [1 g Mg=83.3 mEq or 41.1 mmol] Magnesium oxide, Mag-200 400 mg tablets, Mag-Ox 400 400 mg (241.3 mg Mg) tablets, Almora, Magonate 500 mg Mg gluconate (27 mg Mg) tablets, Magtrate 500 mg Mg gluconate (29 mg Mg) tablets, Chelated Magnesium 500 mg Mg amino acids chelate (100 mg Mg) tablets, Slow-Mag 535 mg $MgCl_2$ (64 mg Mg) tablets, Uro-Mag 140 mg MgO (84.5 mg Mg) capsules, Magonate 54 mg/5 ml Mg as gluconate liquid **Males=350-400 mg/day** **Females=280-300 mg/day**	Maintenance of electrical operations of nerves, muscles, and for the function of enzymes, making of new proteins and storage and release of energy.
Manganese	Manganese sulfate (Chelated) 20, 50 mg tablets: **Dose: 20-50 mg/day**	Enzyme co-factor in protein and energy metabolism. Bone growth and development. Reproduction.
Molybdenum	Sodium molybdate, Ammonium molybdate: **Dose: 20-120 mcg/day**	Enzyme co-factor. Fat and protein metabolism.
Phosphorus	Calcium phosphate, Neutra-Phos Powder, Neutra-Phos-K Capsules, Neutra-Phos-K Powder	Cell membrane and nervous system function. Energy exchange in the body.

Table 11j

VITAMINS AND MINERALS

MINERALS AND TRACE ELEMENTS	NAME	USE OR INDICATION
Potassium	Potassium chloride, Potassium gluconate 500 mg (83.45 mg K) tablets, Potassium gluconate 595 mg (99 mg K) tablets: **Dose: 40-150 mEq/day**	Essential electrolyte. Controls electrical activity of the heart, muscles and nervous system. Regulation of acid-balance (with Na and other electrolytes).
Selenium	Sodium selenate: **Dose: 20-40 mcg/day**	Enzyme co-factor for protection of vital parts of cells against damage by oxidation (e.g., skin, hair, heart muscle). May somehow strengthen the immune system and protect against cancer and heart disease.
Zinc	**Zinc sulfate, 23% Zinc:** Zinc 15 66 mg (15 mg zinc) tablets, Orazinc 110 mg (25 mg zinc) tablets Zinc sulfate 200 mg (45 mg zinc) tablets, Zinc sulfate 220 mg (50 mg zinc), Zinc sulfate, Orazinc, Verazinc, Zinc-220, Zincate 220 mg (50 mg zinc) capsules, **Zinc Gluconate, 14.3% Zinc:** Zinc gluconate 10, 15, 50, 78 mg (1.4, 2, 7, 11 mg Zn resp.) Complex Zinc Carbonates 15 mg/ml liquid **Dose: 1-2 tablets/cap qhs with full glass of water**	Enzyme co-factor. Deficiency will result in loss of appetite, failure to grow, skin changes, slow wound healing, and decreased taste.
Megavitamins		There is No evidence to indicate that large doses of vitamins ensure good health. Some serious side effects have been reported.

48

Table 12

INFANT FORMULAS

Standard Formulas	Sources of Protein	Counseling Guidelines
Breast milk Enfamil Similac SMA Iron-Fortified	human milk cow's milk cow's milk demineralized whey	**Medications to avoid while breast feeding:** bromocriptine cimetidine
Therapeutic Formulas		cyclophosphamide
Milk Allergy		cyclosporine
Isomil ProSobee Nutamigen Nursoy Soyalac	soy isolate soy isolate hydrolyzed casein soy isolate soy extract	doxorubicin ergotamul lithium
Electrolyte Imbalance		methotrexate
Pedialyte Imbalance Pedialyte RS	none none	all drugs of abuse
High Protein and/Or Caloric Requirement		**Consult with pharmacist to thoroughly review all your medications to avoid potential problems.**
Enfamil Premature Formula Similac PM 60/40	cow's milk demineralized whey, casein	

Table 13

ENTERAL NUTRITION PRODUCTS

Food Supplement Products	Dosage Form	Indicated Use
Amin-Aid	powder	nitrogen-restricted diets
Casec	powder	sodium restriction/cholesterol restriction
Controlyte	powder	protein restriction/electrolyte restriction
Enrich	liquid	high-calorie dietary supplement
Ensure	liquid	full liquid diet/liquid supplement/tube feeding
Ensure Plus	liquid	high-calorie liquid food
Gevral Protein	powder	supplementary nourishment
Hepatic-Aid	powder	nutritional deficiencies form chronic liver failure
Instant Breakfast	powder	supplementary nourishment
Isocal	liquid	supplementary nourishment/tube feeding
Osmolite	liquid	tube feeding
Precision High Nitrogen Diet	powder	low residue/high protein requirement/oral tube feeding
Pulmocare	liquid	Pulmonary disease
Scott's Emulsion	liquid	tonic food supplement
Sustacal	liquid	supplementary nourishment
Vital HN	powder	oral or tube feeding/peptide elemental diet

DIABETES CARE PRODUCTS

Products	Counseling Guidelines
1. **Insulin** (See Table 14b) - Insulin lowers blood sugar levels	1. Avoid products containing sugar
2. **Glucagon** - Glucagon used to treat hypoglycemia	2. Good foot care is important
3. **Syringes** - Syringes are used to administer insulin or glucagon	3. Know the symptoms of hypoglycemia and hyperglycemia which include increased heart rate (tachycardia), sweating (diaphoresis), and confusion.
4. **Urine and Blood Glucose Test Products** (See Table 14d) - To test glucose levels in urine and blood	4. Regular exercise is necessary
5. **Glucometers** (See Table 14c) - Glucometers are used to read blood glucose levels	5. Eat a balanced diet
6. **Identification Tags** - Tags are worn by patients to indicate the patient is a diabetic	

Table 14b

INSULINS AVAILABLE IN THE USA

Type (Injection: 100 units/ml)	Animal Source/Brand Name	Manufacturer	Onset of Action Peak/Duration (Hrs)
Short-Acting **Regular** Standard Purified Human	Beef/Pork [Regular Iletin I] Pork [Regular Insulin] Beef [Beef Regular Iletin II] Pork [Regular Purified Pork Iletin II] Pork [Velosulin] - Phosphate Buffer Recombinant DNA [Humulin R & Humulin BR] ("Buffered Regular." Phosphate buffered for pump use. Semi-synthetic [Novolin R] Semi-synthetic [Velosulin Human] (Both also available in cartridge for use in Novopen)	Lilly Sqibb/Novo Lilly Lilly Nordisk-USA Lilly Squibb-Novo Nordisk	1/2-1/2-4/5-7
Short-Acting **Semilente** (Insulin Zinc suspension, prompt) Standard Purified	Beef/Pork [Semilente Iletin I] Pork [Semilente Insulin] Pork [Semilente Purified Pork]	Lilly Sqibb-Novo Squibb-Novo	1-2/4-6/12-16

52

INSULINS AVAILABLE IN THE USA

Type (Injection: 100 units/ml)	Animal Source/Brand Name	Manufacturer	Onset of Action/ Duration (Hrs)
Intermediate-Acting NPH (Isophane Insulin Suspension)			1-2/6-14/24+
Standard	Beef/Pork [NPH Iletin I]	Lilly	
	Beef [NPH Insulin]	Squibb-Novo	
Purified	Beef[Beef NPH Iletin II]	Lilly	
	Pork [Pork NPH Iletin II]	Lilly	
	Pork [NPH Purified Pork]	Squibb-Novo	
	Pork [Insulatard NPH]-Phosphate Buffer	Nordisk	
Human	Recombinant DNA [Humulin N]	Lilly	
	Semi-synthetic [Novolin N]	Squibb-Novo	
	Semi-synthetic [Insulatard NPH]	Nordisk USA	
Lente (Insulin Zn Suspension)			1-3/6-14/24+
Standard	Beef/Pork [Lente Iletin I]	Lilly	
	Beef [Lente Insulin]	Squibb-Novo	
Purified	Beef [Lente Iletin II]	Lilly	
	Pork [Lente Iletin II]	Lilly	
	Pork [Lente Purified Pork]	Squibb-Novo	
Human	Recombinant DNA [Humulin L]	Lilly	
	Semi-synthetic [Novolin L]	Squibb-Novo	
NPH/Regular Mixtures (70%/30%)			
Purified	Pork [Mixtard]	Nordisk-USA	
Human	Recombinant DNA [Mixtard Human 70/30]	Lilly	
	Semi-synthetic [Novolin 70/30]	Squibb-Novo	
	Semi-synthetic [Human mixtard]	Nordisk	

Table 14d

INSULINS AVAILABLE IN THE USA

Type (Injection: 100 units/ml)	Animal Source/Brand Name	Manufacturer	Onset of Action/ Peak/Duration (Hrs)
Long-Acting PZI (Protamine Zn Insulin)	Beef/Pork [Protamine, Zinc & Iletin I]	Lilly Lilly Lilly	6-8/14-24/36+
Standard	Beef [Protamine, Zinc & Iletin II (Beef)] Pork [Protamine, Zinc & Iletin II (Pork)]		
Purified			
Ultralente (Insulin Zn Suspension, Extended) Standard	Beef/Pork [Ultralente Iletin I] Beef [Ultralente Insulin]	Lilly Squibb-Novo	6/18-24/36+
Purified	Beef [Ultralente Purified Beef]	Squibb-Novo	
Human	Biosynthetic [Humulin U]	Lilly	

54

BLOOD GLUCOSE REFLECTANCE METERS

Meter	Blood Glucose Range (mg/dL)	Strip	Counseling Guidelines
Accu-Chek II	20-500	Chemstrip bG	Most "forgiving" of poor technique. Takes 2 minutes. Calibration difficult for some patients. Available in pharmacies.
Diascan S	10-600	Diascan Strips	Easy calibration. Takes 90 seconds. Stores ten readings. Meter operates only between 50-90°F.
Direct 30/30		None	Uses no strip. Replaceable cartridge can be used for unlimited testing for 30 days. Takes 30 seconds. Requires small blood sample. Must be cleansed after use.
ExacTech		ExacTech Strip	Takes 30 seconds. Easy to calibrate. Pen size. Machine reads electreical micro currents formed by interaction between glucose and chemical impregnated on stripe.
Glucometer II Glucometer M	40-400	Glucostrix	Very fast (50 seconds), but very technique dependent. Calibration simple. Difficult for patients lack manual dexterity. Large pad requires more blood than most strips. Glucometer with memory stores up to 26 readings. Glucometer M stores 338 readings which can be interfaced with an IBM data management program. Available in pharmacies.
Glucoscan Glucoscan 3000 with Memory	25-450	Glucoscan strips	Factory calibrated. Stores 29 tests. Takes 60 seconds. Interfaces with a data management program.
One-Touch	0-600	One-Touch strips	Practically technique free. Timing is taken out of patient's hands. Requires only a small amount of blood for testing. Holds 250 readings and can be interfaced with a data manager. Works poorly in bright light.
Tracer		Tracer bG strips	Stores 7 readings. Small size; portable. Small strips require smaller volumes of blood for testing.

BLOOD GLUCOSE REAGENT STRIPS AVAILABLE IN PHARMACIES

Product	Blood Glucose Range (mg/dL)	Counseling Guidelines
Chemstrips	20-800	May be read visually or with a meter: Accu-Chek II or Glucochek II bG. Developed strip is stable for one week if stored in the bottle with a dessicant.
Glucostix	20-800	May be read visually or with a meter: Glucometer II.
Visidex	20-800	May be read visually only.

URINE GLUCOSE TESTS

Test	Counseling Guidelines
Copper Reduction Method: Clinitest	Less specific for glucose, but it is more quantitative, especially for larger amounts of glucose in the urine. Now rarely used. Less sensitive than the glucose oxidase method, often giving false-negative values at very low glucose concentrations. This is a particular disadvantage for non-insulin-dependent patients in whom aglycosuria is a goal.
Glucose Oxidase Methods:	More specific for glucose than Clinitest, but are less quantitative. More sensitive to glucose at low concentrations but false-low readings can occur at high glucose concentrations and in the presence of ketones.
1. Tes-Tape	Too sensitive, resulting in positive reactions to urine samples which contain little or no glucose.
2. Diastix	More accurate and has a color chart that is more quantitative than Tes-Tape.
3. Chemstrip uG	Several advantages over the other products: As accurate as Diastix. Compares favorably with Clinistix. Its main disadvantage is that it requires two minutes for completion of the enzymatic reaction. While Diastix may read too low in the high range, Chemstrip uG tends to read too high.
Urine Glucose Tests which also test for Ketones 1. Keto-Diastix 2. Chemstrips uGK	

DRUG INTERFERENCE WITH URINE GLUCOSE TESTS

Group A: Drugs that interfere with urine glucose tests - Avoid prior to test.	Group B: Drugs that may interfere with urine glucose tests - Avoid prior to test.	Group C: Drugs that *do not* interfere with urine glucose tests
1. Ascorbic acid 2. Beta-Lactam antibiotics 3. Cephalosporins 4. Penicillins 5. Monobactams (aztreonam) 6. Carbapenems (imipenem) 7. Levodopa 8. Salicylates	1. Chloral Hydrate 2. Hyaluronidase 3. Nalidixic acid 4. Nitrofurantoin 5. p-Aminosalicylic acid 6. Phenazopyridine 7. Probenecid 8. x-ray contrast media	1. Aminoglycoside antibiotics 2. Chloramphenicol 3. Ciprofloxacin 4. Ephedrine 5. Epinephrine 6. Ethacrynic Acid 7. Indomethacin 8. Isoniazid (INH) 9. Lincomycin 10. Methenamine 11. Methyldopa 12. Metaproterenol 13. Morphine 14. Nicotinic acid 15. Phenothiazines 16. Sulfonamide antibiotics 17. Tetracycline antibiotics (may contain ascorbic acid) 18. Thiazide diuretics

Table 15

OPHTHALMIC DRUGS

Decongestants and Vasoconstrictors	Counseling Guidelines
Phenylephrine [**Prefrin Liquifilm**]	Decongestants and vasoconstrictors are used to "get the red out" and relieve minor eye symptoms such as burning, stinging, itching, tearing, tiredness or eye strain. OcuHist, an antihistamine ophthalmic product temporarily relieves itching and redness of the eye caused by pollen, ragweed, grass, animal hair, and dander according to manufacturer Pfizer.
Naphazoline [**Bausch & Lomb Allergy Drops**]	They are not recommended for long term use
Tetrahydrozoline [**Murine Plus, Visine Allergy, Visine Moisturizer**]	Eye washes are used to remove a foreign particle from the eye Patients with Glaucoma should consult a physician before using any eye products
Naphazoline HCL 0.025%+Pheniramine maleate 0.3% [**OcuHist**] (*Formerly AK-Con-A^R , Rx by Akorn*)	Wash hands before administration
Artificial Tear Solutions	Keep the lenses clean on a daily basis with the use of a cleaning solution
Viscosity agent (polyvinyl alcohol, hydroxyethycellulose) [**Akwa Tears, Tear Drop, Puralube Tears, LubriTears, Dry Eyes**, etc.]	Contact lenses should be kept in a soaking solution when they are not in the eye
	A Wetting Agent should be used to put the contact lens in the eye
Preservatives (edetate disodium, thimerosal, benzalkonium chloride,chlorobutanol)	Always wash hands before handling the contact lenses
Eye Wash Products or irrigating Solutions	Never administer eye drops to the eyes while contacts are in place
Buffers (sodium phosphate, boric acid, NaCl, KCL, etc) [**Eye Wash, AK-Rinse, Blinx, Optigene, Visual-Eyes**]	Use hair and deodorant sprays before the lenses are put in place
	Sterilization of soft contact lenses by thermal (Saline solution + heat) and chemical (Bactericidal solution) methods.

Table 16

OTIC PRODUCTS

Causes of Ear Discomfort	Counseling Guidelines

1. Ear wax build-up
 	
Treatment:
1a. Carbamide peroxide (urea peroxide) in **Murine Ear** Wax Removal Systems, **Debrox** Drops, Ear Drops by Murine
  b. Warm Olive Oil
 	
2. Swimmer's Ear
 	
Treatment:
2a. Anhydrous glycerin in isopropyl alcohol (**Swim Ear**)
  b. Ear plugs
	Do not put anything in an ear canal if there is drainage (such as pus or blood).
	
	Do not stick things in the ear to break up the earwax.
	
	If not better in two days, or worse, contact a physician.

Table 17

MEDICAL & HEALTH SUPPLIES

Health Supplies	Counseling Guidelines
Ambulatory Aids Canes Crutches, Walker, and Wheelchairs	Consult with pharmacist and/or follow package insert directions. Carry cane on strong side.
Respiratory Therapy Instruments (Asthma & COPD): Peak Expiratory Flow Rate (PEFR) Meters Metered Dose Inhalers (MDI) and Dry Powder Inhalers (DPI) Extension devices (Spacers) [Inspirease^R, Inhal-Aid^R] Nebulizers Humidifiers & Vaporizers	If using only one crutch, hold it on side opposite weak leg. If two crutches, step forward with right leg and left crutch, followed by left leg and right crutch, and so on. Proper use of respiratory therapy instruments will ensure beneficialeffects and avoidance of adverse effects. Consult your pharmacist or physician for advice and instructions.
Diagnostic Products: Urine Nicotine & Byproducts Test [NicCheck I] Home Cholesterol Test Kits [Cholestrak™] Home Blood Pressure (BP) Monitoring Device (with Cuff and Meter) Home Fecal (stool) occult test kits [EZ- Detect ^R] Home Glucose Monitoring kit (See Diabetes Care) Hypodermic Equipment & Care: **Care of Hypodermic Equipment:** **Stain Removal:** Hot Conc. Alkaline Solutions (KOH, NaOH); **Kill Microorganisms:** Sterilization . **Blood Stains Removal:** Enzyme Preparations, Conc. Ammonia,10% HNO$_3$, Citric acid. Home Ovulation Prediction and Pregnancy Test Kits [various] Home HIV Detection Kits [Confide^R, Home Access^R]*	NicCheck I is a white strip that detects the presence of nicotine in the urine of a smoker. Check self-testing kits for expiration dates Ambulatory cholesterol monitoring can also lead to early detection of high and low cholesterol and prevention of coronary artery disease heart) complications and other problems associated with too low levels of cholesterol. Ambulatory BP monitoring can lead to early detection of elevated BP and prevention of complications. Regular fecal (stool) testing can lead to early detection of colorectal cancer and prevention of consequences. Early detection of elevated blood glucose will avoid diabetic complications. *Early detection of pregnancy can help in family planning.* *Early detection of HIV infection can lead to early interventions.* **Confide, removed from the market for lack of consumer demand.*

Table 18

CONTRACEPTIVE AIDS

Products	Spermicides	General Information

1. **Spermicides**
   Delfen **(foam)**
   Encare **(suppository)**
   Semicid **(suppository)**
 	
2. **Spermicides Used With A Diaphragm**
   Gynol **(jelly)**
   Ortho-Cream **(cream)**
	1. Nonoxynol-9
	2. Octoxynol
	3. Menfegol
		1. **Douching** should not be used for contraception.
		
		2. **Condoms** protect against pregnancy and against sexually transmitted diseases (STDs).
		
		3. Never use Vaseline or any other petroleum product on condoms. If lubrication is needed, use a water soluble lubricant such as **K-Y Jelly.**

Table 19

PERSONAL CARE PRODUCTS

Product	Active Ingredient	Use
1. Betadine Douche	Povidine - iodine	bacterial infection
2. Massengill Douche	Cetylpyridinium chloride imidazolidinyl urea	cleaning
3. Norforms	Methylbenzethonium chloride	reduce or mask odor
4. Feminine Deodorant Sprays		reduce or mask odor reduce or mask pain
5. Gyne-Lotrimin Vaginal Inserts	Clotrimazole	yeast infections
6. Monistat-3 vaginal cream	Miconazole	yeast infections x 3 days
7. Monistat - 7 vaginal Cream	Miconazole	yeast infections x 7 days
8. Femstat-3 vaginal cream 2%	Butoconazole nitrate	yeast infections
9. Vagistat-1	Tioconazole	yeast infection (vaginal candidiasis):
		1-Dose treatment
10. Advil, Nuprin, Motrin IB	Ibuprofen	menstrual pain
11. Tylenol	Acetaminophen	menstrual pain
12. Sanitary Napkins/Tampons		menstrual periods

Counseling Guidelines

Avoid douches during pregnancy.
Always use good personal hygiene.
Allergic sensitivity or contact irritation can occur with some products.
Use tampons with the minimum absorbency needed to control menstrual flow,
in order to reduce the risk of Toxic Shock Syndrome (TSS).

DENTAL AND MOUTH CARE

Products	General Information
1. **Toothbrushes**	1. Use a soft to medium nylon bristle toothbrush and replace every 2-3 months. (Crest Complete) Use 2-3 times daily after every meal. Other types of brushes include the Electronic (Broxodent), Pediatric, and Children's toothbrushes.
2. **Toothpastes (Dentifrices)** -Forms: Gels, Pastes, and Powders.	
3. **Dental floss**	
4. **Mouthwashes** Temporary bactericidals. All types have equal effects. Used for freshening and cleaning mouth. **Components** (sweetener, astringent, demulcent, detergent, germicidal agents, anesthetic, analgesic, preservatives...etc) E.g., 1. Listerine 2. Hydrogen peroxide (concentration reduced to 50%) - works by releasing oxygen free radicals (charged molecules) to dislodge debris from tissues (wounds, areas).	2. Use a toothpaste accepted by the American Dental Association (ADA)(e.g; Aquafresh, Colgate, Sensodyne, Tartar Control Crest). 3. Dental floss is essential for removing plaque and debris. Use about 18 inches of floss and wrap most of it around a middle finger. 4. Mouthwashes that contain Phenol (ex. Chloraseptic) are used to treat a sore throat 5. Visit your dentist regularly.

DENTAL AND MOUTH CARE

Products	General Information
5. **Denture Products** 1. Regular toothpaste - Use normal dentifrices. 2. Alkaline Hypochlorite Bleach (alkaline peroxides) - Cleans dentures by dissolving mucin. Kills bacteria and fungi (bactericidal/fungicidal). 3. Denture Adherents and Liners - See Dentist for proper fitting. 4. Denture Repair Kits - Acrylic materials/glue. **Should NOT be stocked by Pharmacist.** 5. Ultrasonic Unit - Used to clean dentures. Expensive. 6. **Fever blisters** 7. **Canker/Cold Sores Products** Anesthetic products containing benzocaine 5-20%, benzyl alcohol 0.05-0.1%, menthol 0.04-2%, phenolate sodium 0.5-1.5% phenol, dyclonine 0.05-0.1%, hexyresorcinol 0.05-0.1%, phenol 0.05-1.5%, salicyl alcohol 1-6%. Temporary relief of cold sores. 8. **Toothache medicines**	5. Brush dentures at least once daily. Dentures should be rinsed properly before insertion in the mouthafter cleansing. Cleansing solutions may be toxic to mouth gums and to children. Keep out of reach of children (locked). 6. Fever blisters must run its course (7-10 days) 7. Canker sores can be treated with **Oragel** or Orabase with benzocaine, Orabase with hydrocortisone and Peroxide gels. Benzocaine can cause allergic reactions resulting in itching and burning. Chronic use may cause hepatotoxicity (liver dysfunction). 8. Never apply **aspirin** directly to the teeth or gums (Irritation/Bleeding). Note: Drugs known to cause oral problems: 1. Anticholinergics (e.g., benztropine [Cogentin]) 2. Drugs with anticholinergic side effects (antipsychotics, antihistamines, antidepressants-TCAs) 3. Phenytoin (Dilantin) - Gingival hyperplasia 4. Tetracycline - superinfection/stains teeth-green, gold, or brown in children 5. Other broadspectrum antibiotics & Chloramphenicol - superinfection 6. Drugs that cause dysguesia (taste sensation changes) 7. Cigarettes/tobacco 8. Corticosteroids - superinfection due to immunosuppression 9. Chemotherapeutic,antineuplastic agents - stomatitis, superinfection - Use Mycelex, Nystatin ...etc

Table 21a

DERMATOLOGICAL PRODUCTS

Topical Preparations	Counseling Guidelines
1. **Acne** Benzoyl Peroxide [Desquam-X, Neutrogena, Clearasil, Ambi-10] 2. **Sunscreens** Para-Aminobenzoic Acid (PABA)	1. Never pick or squeeze acne. 2. Wear a sunscreen with a **Sun Protection Factor** (SPF) of 15 or higher. Avoid sunning between 10 a.m. thru 2 p.m. when sun rays are most damaging. Submerge burned area in cold water.
3. **Poison Ivy** Benzocaine Calamine lotion Aveeno Colloidal Oatmeal 4. **Insect repellents** [Off] **Bee and wasp Stings** Benzocaine Epinephrine 0.15 mg IM [EpiPen Auto-Injector] - Rx/OTC 5. **Head Lice** Permethril 1% [**Nix**ᴿ] 6. **Hair Regrowth Products** Minoxidil 2% solution [Rogaineᴿ] Minoxidil ES [Rogaine ESᴿ]	3. If poison ivy is severe, in eyes or genitals - contact physician. 4. Remove stinger from bee bite, do not squeeze the stinger. 5. Sterilize all personal clothing, bed clothes and bedding of the lice infested person in hot water. Wash all personal articles such as combs and brushes in hot water 6. Rogaine is indicated for male-pattern baldness. Consult your pharmacist or physician for directions, Rogaine ES for men will grow up to 46% more hair than regular. Rogaine, with the onset of hair regrowth occurring at 8 weeks (Regular Rogaine at 16 weeks).

DERMATOLOGICAL PRODUCTS

7. **Dandruff** (Chronic noninflammatory scalp condition that results from excessive scaling of scalp epidermis. Pruritus/itching is common). **Pyrithione zinc shampoo 1-2%** [Danex, Zincon, Head & Shoulders, DHS Zinc, Sebulon, Theraplex Z, ZNP Bar (soap)] **Selenium sulfide shampoo 1-2.5%** [Selsun Blue, Head & Shoulders] **Coal Tar Shampoo 1-10%** [DHS Tar, Doctar, Theraplex T, Zetar, Ionil.T Plus, Neutragena T/Gel, Pentrax, Tegrin Medicated, Denorex, Duplex T, Iocon, Polytar] **Keratolytic shampoo (Salicylic acid or Sulfur)**	Washing the hair and scalp with nonmedicated shampoo every other day or even daily is often sufficient to control dandruff. If it is not, then use medicated shampoo. Allow the medicated shampoo to remain on the hair for approximately 1 minute before thorough rinsing. Discoloration of light hair, clothing, and jewelry may occur with use of coal tar-containing shampoos. If the condition worsens or if symptoms persist for more than 7 days, consult a physician or pharmacist. Avoid use for children under 2 years of age, except under the advice and supervision of a physician.

DERMATOLOGICAL PRODUCTS

8. **Seborrheic Dermatitis (Seborrhea)** {Patchy inflammatory head, scalp and trunk condition characterized by yellowish-red lesions, oily-appearing, yellowish scales. Pruritus is common. It may be an extension of dandruff}. **Pyrithione Zinc shampoo** **Selenium sulfide shampoo** **Coal Tar shampoo 5%** **Hydrocortisone lotion** (corticosteroid)	
9. **Eczema (Atopic Dermatitis)** {Skin condition characterized by intense itching that is often intermittent, leading to vigorous itch-scratch cycles. Inflammation and scaling may occur. May be associated with various factors, such as irritants, allergens, extremes of temperature and humidity, dry skin, emotional stress, and cutaneous infections}. **Diphenhydramine (Benadryl, Various)** {Antihistamines} topical/systemic	Maintaining skin hydration with products such as soaps (e.g., Cetaphil), tepid water containing colloidal oatmeal, and petrolatum ointments, may decrease itching.

Table 22

OSTOMY CARE PRODUCTS

Products	General Infomation
1. Ostomy Adhesive Disk 2. Ostomy Cementof adhesive tape 3. Ostomy Solvent 4. Ostomy Deodorizer 5. Ostomy Skin Protective	1. Adhesive disk attaches the appliance to the skin 2. Cement holds the appliance to the skin 3. Solvents help to remove an appliance, to remove excess glue from the skin, and to clean the face plate 4. Deodorizers are used to mask odor 5. Skin protectives act as a chemical bandage that aids in the removal of adhesive tape.

Table 23

FOOT CARE PRODUCTS

Foot Condition and Treatment	Athlete's Foot Patient Consultation
1. **Foot Odor** Doctor Scholl's Odor Attackers Baking Soda	1. Do not expect dramatic remission of the condition. If no improvement in 4 weeks, consult a physician
2. **Athlete's Foot** (Tinea pedis) Aluminum acetate [Burow's solution/ Dome boro] Aluminum chloride Clotrimazole [**Lotrimin Antifungal-AF**, Mycelex Solution] Miconazole [Micatin] Tolnaftate [Tinactin, NP-27] Undecylenic acid and zinc unde-cylenate [Desenex]	2. Discontinue the product if itching,swelling, or exacerbation of the disease occurs. Wash hands thoroughly after applying product. 3. Have good foot hygiene; clean and thoroughly dry daily
3. **Jockitch** (Tinea Cruris) Antifungal powders [Tinactin]	
4. **Callus/Corn/Wart** Salicylic acid [Wart-Off, Compound-W]	

Table 24a

ADULT URINARY INCONTINENCE (UI)PRODUCTS

Products	Description	Counseling Guidelines
I. Stayfree Serenity	1. Bladder protection pads $4.32 20 ct. 2. Bladder protection guards $17.28 30 ct. 3. Super plus absorbency guards $16.98 24ct 4. regular absorbency $16.98 36 ct. Distributed by: **McNeil-PPC, Inc.** **(Johnson & Johnson) Skillman. NJ 08558**	1. Require referrals for medical evaluation because UI is a symptom and not a single disease process. 2. Prophylactic program and recommendation of therapy for uncomplicated, uninfected cases of diaper rash (dermatitis), prickly heat, and adult incontinence (e.g., frequent diaper changes, frequent exposure to air, and application of a protectant such as **zinc oxide paste**).
II. Fresh n'Gentle	1. Extra absorbency $10.53 30 ct. 2. Fitted briefs $10.53 30 ct. Distributed by: **Winn Dixie Stores Inc.** Jacksonville, FL 32203	3. Medication counseling on the complications and assistance in selecting appropriate absorbent devices for persons with urinary incontinence.
III. Poise Guards (Depend)	1. Extra absorbency $4.17 20 ct. 2. Extra plus absorbency $15.48 30 ct. 3. Super absorbency $15.48 30 ct. 4. Super plus absorbency $15.48 30 ct Distributed by: **Kimberly-Clark, Corp.** Neenah, WI 54956	4. Use OTC chlorophyll [e.g., **Derifil, Pals,** and **Nullo**] to decrease embarassing odor due to UI. 5. Require referrals for medical management of pressure ulcers (decubiti) associated with UI. 6. Decongestants (e.g., ephedrine, pseudoephedrine, phenyleph-rine, and phenylpropanolamine) may be recommended because they cause urinary retention by stimulating alpha and beta receptors, which enhances bladder filling and increases bladder sphincter tone.

ADULT URINARY INCONTINENCE (UI) PRODUCTS

Products	Description	Counseling Guidelines
IV. Depend	1. Extra absorbency $15.38 34 ct. 2. Depend overnight $15.38 20 ct. 3. Non-elastic leg extra absorbency undergarments $15.38 30 ct. 4. Easy-fit $15.38 28 ct. 5. Fitted briefs $15.38 22 ct. 6. Underpads bedsize $6.38 18 ct. 7. Guards for men $5.96 18 ct. Distributed by: **Kimberly-Clark Corp.** P.O. Box 2020, Neenah, WI 54957-2020	7. Alpha-receptor agonists used for hypertension treatment may also enhance the action of adrenergic receptors in the bladder. 8. Diuretics, taken late in the evening, may cause or worsen UI; and sedatives/hypnotics may decrease the older patient's awareness of bladder filling. 9. Drugs with anticholinergic action (phenothiazines, antihistamines, antidepressants) may inhibit bladder function (emptying). Ask pharmacists for side effects and contraindications of these medications.
V. Attend	1. Undergarments with belts/super absorbency $12.98 30ct. 2. Guards/super absorbency $9.68 28ct. 3. Pads light bladder protection $4.77 22ct. Distributed by: **Procter & Gamble**, Cincinnati, OH 45202	10. Prescription medications such as Oxybutynin chloride, flavoxate hydrochloride, or hyoscyamine may be initiated by physician. Consult your pharmacist for drug information. 11. Consult pharmacist for use of protective undergarments, and pads (absorbent products) aimed at protecting clothing, bedding, and furniture while allowing independence and mobility.

ADULT INCONTINENCE (UI) PRODUCTS

Products	Description	Counseling Guidelines
VI. Reliance = Rx	Urinary control insert for women as an alternative to adult diapers. In trials, Reliance controlled urine loss in 95% of patients studied. Nearly all patients reported improved quality of life. Available in 5 lengths through prescription.	12. Pharmacist will counsel patient regarding embarrassment, depression, low self-esteem, social isolation, decreased intimate contact and sexual activity, pressure ulcers and skin irritation. 13. Dehydration and hypotension may be associated with fluid intake restriction in an attempt to limit episodes of urinary frequency. Consult the pharmacist. 14. Other causes of UI include but are not limited to impaired cognitive function or perception, stroke, diminished mobility, environmental barriers, anatomical and physiologic dysfunction, and psychologic unwillingness to toilet in the proper place.
	Note: All above prices are according to Winn Dixie Supermarket's price.	15. UI may also result from the medical use of physical restraints that make toileting without assistance impossible.

HERBS & PHYTOMEDICINAL AGENTS

Products: Common Name/Scientific Name	Description/Claimed Indications	Counseling Guidelines
GASTROINTESTINAL DISORDERS: I. **Nausea & Vomiting (Motion Sickness)** **Ginger** [*Zingiber officinale*] 500 mg capsules Dose: 2-4 gm/day	Carminative (antiflatulent, anti-colic), antiemetic (nausea/vomiting or motion sickness), cholagogue, positive inotropic. **Indication:** Dyspepsia, colic, prophylactic relief of symptoms of motion sickness.	Avoid in treatment of postoperative nausea. Contraindicated in gallstone pain and nausea associated with pregnancy. Take 1 capsule 30 minutes prior to travel departure, then 1-2 capsules every 4 hours.
II. **Constipation** A. **Bulk-Producing Laxatives** **Plantago Seed & Husk** [*Plantago psyllium*] {Plantain or psyllium seed}, Dose: 7.5 gm (Average 4-20 gm/day)	Bulk-forming laxatives; for treatment of chronic constipation and conditions necessitating soft stools, such as hemorrhoids, anal fissures, rectal-anal surgery, total cholesterol (TC) and low density lipoprotein (LDL) lowering efficacy.	Take with plenty (at least 150 ml) of water, 30-60 minutes after meals or the administration of other drugs.
B. **Stimulant Laxatives** 1. **Significant Stimulant Laxative Senna** [*Senna alexandrina*] 2 gm **Cascara Sagrada Buckthorn (Frangula) Bark** 2. **Other Stimulant Laxatives Aloe (Aloes) Rhubarb**	Cathartic for treatment of constipation.	Cramping discomfort may occur. Potassium/electrolyte/fluid imbalances may occur. Not recommended in concurrent digoxin and antiarrhythmic drugs use. Not recommended during pregnancy or lactation. Generally safe.

<u>Disclaimer:</u> The claimed indications have NOT been evaluated by the FDA. The products are not intended to diagnose, treat, cure, or prevent any disease. The FDA has not received sufficient data to permit these products to be placed in Category I. These products are sold in the United States not as drugs but as dietary supplements. Some of these agents and/or extracts are already FDA-approved and are available either OTC or by prescription. Consult appropriate references.

Table 25b

HERBS & PHYTOMEDICINAL AGENTS

Products: Common Name/Scientific Name	Description/Claimed Indications	Counseling Guidelines
III. Indigestion - Dyspepsia **A. Carminatives** **1. Significant Carminative Herbs** **Peppermint** [*Menthax piperita*] EC capsules 1.5-3 gm/day or 0.6-1.2 ml EC peppermint oil per day.	Flavoring agents. Treatment of Irritable Bowel Syndrome (IBS) and spastic GI tract complaints.	Generally safe. Allergy (anaphylactic shock) from drinking chamomile tea may occur.

Chamomile [*Chamomile recutita*] Tea (150 ml hot water over 3 gm dried flower heads, steeped for 10 minutes) drunk 3-4 times daily with meals.
 	
2. Minor Carminative Herbs
    Anise
    Caraway
    Coriander
    Fennel
    Calamus
	Antiinflammatory, spasmolytic, and antimicrobial activity. GI spasms, GI tract inflammatory diseases, peptic ulcers, mouthwash for inflammatory conditions of the oral cavity and gums. Topical formulations (creams, ointments) for skin and mucous membrane inflammations and bacterial skin diseases. Wound-healing effects for promotion of granulation and tissue regeneration. Treatment of eczema.	

3. Cholagogues
    Turmeric
    Boldo
    Dandelion
	A cholagogue is a drug which causes an increased flow of bile into the intestine.	

HERBS AND PHYTOMEDICINAL AGENTS

Products: Common Name/Scientific Name	Description/Claimed Indications	Counseling Guidelines
IV. **Hepatotoxicity (Liver Damage)** **Milk Thistle** [*Silybum marianum*] 80 mg, 140 mg capsules/ tablets (Max. dose: 200-420 mg/day or 12-15 gm of seeds per day). Schizandra V. **Gastric & Duodenal (Peptic) Ulcers** **Licorice** [*Glycyrrhiza*, etc.] 5-15 gm powder/day or 200-600 mg of glycyrrhizin X 4-6 weeks. **Ginger** VI. **Diarrhea** **Blackberry Leaves** **Blueberry Leaves** **Raspberry Leaves** **Blackberry Root** **Blueberries** **Bilberries**	Hepatoprotectants by scavenging of free radicals, alteration of the outer liver membrane cell structure to protect liver cells from the entry of toxic substances, stimulation of RNA polymerase, enhancing ribosome protein synthesis, which activates the liver's regenerative capacity through cell development. Used for prophylaxis and treatment of chronic hepatotoxicity (inflammatory liver disorders and cirrhosis resulting from chronic hepatitis or fatty infiltration induced by alcohol or other chemicals). Peptic ulcer disease, antitussive and expectorant (secretolytic) effects. Fifty times sweeter than sugar. **Mechanisms:** Causes increase in prostaglandins in the stomach, thereby producing protective effect on gastric mucosa, resulting in promotion of the healing of gastric ulcers.	Mild transient diarrhea may occur. Duration of therapy should NOT exceed 4-6 weeks. Licorice may cause increase in glucocorticoid and/or mineralocorticoid activities, resulting in sodium retention, potassium excretion, and high blood pressure and potassium loss (hypokalemia). Potassium loss may be increased by concurrent use of thiazide diuretics, resulting in digoxin toxicity. **Do not exceed recommended dose.** Contraindications of licorice include liver cirrhosis, cholestatic liver disease, hypertonia, hypokalemia, and pregnancy. Ginger may interact with blood thinners to cause bleeding. Avoid concurrent use.

HERBS AND PHYTOMEDICINAL AGENTS

Products: Common Name/Scientific Name	Description/Claimed Indications	Counseling Guidelines

VII. Appetite Loss (Anorexia)
A. Significant Bitter Herbs
  Gentian
  Centaury
B. Minor Bitter Herbs
  Bitterstick
  Blessed Thistle
  Bogbean
  Wormwood
		See table 3b for appetite stimulants.

KIDNEY, URINARY URINARY TRACT & PROSTATE DISORDERS:
 	
I. Infections & Kidney Stones
A. Significant Aquaretic-Antiseptic Herbs
Golden rod [*Solidago,* etc.] 6-12 gm 240 ml boiling water over 3-5 gm of herb.
  Parsely
  Juniper
B. Minor Aquaretic Herbs
  Birch Leaves
  Lovage Root
	An aquaretic for use in irrigation therapy against lower urinary tract inflammation, prevention and treatment of urinary calculi and kidney stones.	Allergic reaction may occur.
		
		Contraindicated in edema due to impaired heart or kidney function.
		
		Parely may stimulate the uterine muscle. Avoid during pregnancy.

C. Antiseptic Herbs Bearberry or Uva-ursi [*Arctostaphylos uva-ursi*] 10 gm powder/day or 400-700 mg arbutin X 1 wk Macerate dried cut or powdered herb overnight in 150 ml of cold water.	Antiseptic action. Minimal diuretic activity. Antibacterial activity for urinary tract infections (UTIs).	Requires alkaline pH for activation. Hence, take with foods known to induce alkalinuria (milk, vegetables such as tomatoes and potatoes, fruits, fruit juices. Ingestion of 6-8 gm of sodium bicarbonate a day will also produce alkalinity during treatment. Nausea and vomiting may occur. Use should be limited to 1 week or less.

HERBS & PHYTOMEDICINAL AGENTS

Products: Common Name/Scientific Name	Description/Claimed Indications	Counseling Guidelines
D. Anti-Infective Herbs **Cranberry Juice/Capsules** [Vaccinium macrocarpon] 90 ml = 6 capsules per day as UTI preventive. 360-960 ml daily for UTI treatment. **II. Benign Prostatic Hyperplasia (Prostate Enlargement)** **Saw Palmetto (Sabal)** [*Serenoa repens*] 1-2 gm of the ground, dried fruits or 320 mg of a lipophilic fruit extract daily. **Nettle Root** **Nettle Leaves**	Bacteriostatic effect. Hence, used for prevention and treatment of UTIs. Mechanism: Prevents the adhesion of *E.coli* and other uropathogenic bacteria to the mucosal cells of the urinary tract. Urinary deodorizer secondary to urinary acidification. Therefore, can reduce the urinary odor of incontinent patients. This occurs because it lowers the pH enough to retard the degradation of urine by *E. coli*, which produces the offensive ammoniacal odors. Antiandrogenic (testosterone/ dihydrotesterone reduction) and anti-inflammatory activity as well as antiedematous (inhibition of the arachidonic acid pathway) activity. Used for treatmet of symptoms associated with **benign prostatic hyperplasia** (BPH) {e.g., micturition difficulties and for reduction of prostate enlargement.	Generally safe for prevention of UTIs, but once a UTI has already developed, consult physician for appropriate assessment, cultures and antibiotic selection. Cranberry juice/capsules may interact with pravastatin (Pravachol), a cholesterol-lowering medicine, to cause increased levels of pravastatin. **Note:** Simvastatin (Zocor) and Lovastatin (Mevacor) have been reported to interact with grapefruit juice. Consult your pharmacist. Increased levels of "statins" may result in rhabdomyolysis (muscle pain). **Mechanism:** Inhibition of cytochrome P3A4 enzyme. Consult with patient's Urologist.

HERBS AND PHYTOMEDICINAL AGENTS

Products: Common Name/Scientific Name	Description/Claimed Indications	Counseling Guidelines
RESPIRATORY TRACT DISORDERS: **I. Bronchial Asthma** **Ephedra** [*Ephedra sinica*, etc] 2 gms of the herb in 240 ml of boiling water for 10 minutes = 15-30 mg of ephedrine and drunk as a tea.	Treatment of bronchial asthma via bronchodilation and reductions in bronchial edema (sympathomimetic bronchodilator).	Avoid if suffering from heart conditions, hypertension, diabetes, or thyroid disease. Ephedrine and related alkalloids are CNS stimulants; overdose can result in nervousness, insomnia, and palpitations. Products containing ephedra herb, often spiked with ephedrine and/or pseudoephedrine, are commonly used in weight loss formulations. **No evidence to support safety and effectiveness.**

II.   Colds and Flu
A.   Demulcent Antitussives
    Coltsfoot
    iceland Moss
    Marshmallow Root
    Mullein Flowers
    Plantain Leaves
    Slippery Elm [*Ulmus rubra*]
    0.5-2 gm of powdered bark in 10 parts hot water (5-20 ml). Available in liquids, tablets, and troches.
	Demulcent, emollient, and nutrient (water-soluble polysaccharide, starch) for soothing irritated mucous membranes or ulcerations of the digestive tract, relieving gastritis, colitis, and gastric or duodenal ulcers, and soothing sorethroat.	**Ephedrine-containing products recently banned/removed from OTC market due to use in the manufacture of the illicit drugs methamphetamine and methcathinone.**
		
		Ephedra will increase the effects of monoamine oxidare inhibitors and caffeine.
		
		Ephendra will interact with ephedrine given during surgery following general anesthesia and drop in blood pressure to cause severe increase in blood pressure and stroke. Avoid use prior to surgery.
		
		FDA-approved for use as soothing demulcent for sorethroat. Relatively safe.

HERBS & PHYTOMEDICINAL AGENTS

Products: Common Name/Scientific Name	Description/Claimed Indications	Counseling Guidelines
B. Expectorants 1. Nauseant-Expectorants Ipecac Lobelia 2. Local Irritants Horehound [*Marrubium vulgare*] 0.75 - 1 liters/day 2 gms of the dried herb is steeped in 240 ml of boiling water. Anise Fennel Thyme Eucalyptus Leaves 3. Surface-Tension Modifiers Ivy Primula Licorice (Glycyrrhiza) Senega Snakeroot	Expectorant and antitussive activity. Cough suppressant, digestive aid, and appetite stimulant.	The FDA has declared it ineffective as an OTC cough suppressant and expectorant. See sections on colds, cough suppressants and expectorants.

Table 25g

HERBS AND PHYTOMEDICINAL AGENTS

Products: Common Name/Scientific Name	Description/Claimed Indications	Counseling Guidelines
CARDIOVASCULAR SYSTEM DISORDERS: **I. Angina (Chest Pain)** **Hawthorn** [*Crataegus laevigata*] 3-4 gm of the dried drug in divided doses of 1 gm.	Treatment of diminished cardiac performance (Stages I and II), heart conditions not requiring digitalis, mild and stable angina pectoris, mild dysrhythmia. Flowering tops used in sleep-inducing preparations.	Relatively safe if used under medical supervision.
II. Arterosclerosis **Garlic** [*Allium sativum*] 400-1,200 mg of dried powder/day or, 2-5 gm of the fresh bulb/day equivalent to 4-12 mg of alliin or 2-5 mg of allicin.	Antiplatelet aggregation (antithrombotic) and antimicrobial (antibacterial, antifungal) activity.	May cause GI discomfort and rare allergic reactions. Potentially useful in treatment of high blood pressure, atherosclerosis, hypoglycemia, digestive ailments, colds, flu, and bronchitis. **More data is needed to substantiate effectiveness.** Garlic may interact with blood thinners to cause bleeding.
III. Peripheral Vascular Disease **A. Cerebrovascular Disease** **Ginkgo** [*Ginkgo biloba*] 120-160 mg of leaf extract/day X 4-6 weeks.	Vasodilatory activity. Causes increase in peripheral blood flow rate. Useful in varicose conditions, post-thrombotic syndrome, chronic cerebral vascular insufficiency, short-term memory loss, cognitive disorders secondary to depression, dementia, tinnitus, vertigo, and obliterative arterial disease of the lower limbs.	Generally safe. Rare side effects including headache, dizziness, and vertigo, minor GI disturbances. Ginkgo may interact with blood thinners to cause bleeding. It may also interact with vitamin E to increase bleeding risk. Avoid concurrent use.

HERBS & PHYTOMEDICINAL AGENTS

Products: Common Name/Scientific Name	Description/Claimed Indications	Counseling Guidelines

CARDIOVASCULAR SYSTEM DISORDERS (Continued)
B. Other Peripheral Arterial Circulation Disorders
     Rosemary
C. Venous Disorders
1. Varicose Vein Syndrome
     Horse Chestnut Seed
     Butcher's-Broom		

D. Cardiotoxicity (Cardiac Damage)
     Grapeseed and/or Pinebark
     [Vitis vinifera]
     75-300 mg/day X 3 weeks,
     then 40-80 mg/day
     maintenance dose.
	Antioxidant, for treatment of circulatory disorders such as hypoxia from atherosclerosis, inflammation, and cardiac or cerebral infarction.	Generally safe.

IV. Congestive Heart Failure (CHF)
     Herbs Containing Potent Cardioactive Glycosides:
     Digitalis
     Digitalis Lanata
     Adonis
     Apocynum (Black Indian Hemp)
     Black Hellebore
     Cactus Grandiflorus,
     Convallaria (Lily-of-the-Valley)
     Oleander
     Squill
     Strophanthus
	Digitalis is the precursor of **digoxin** which is a popular prescription medication for the treatment of congestive heart disease.	Consult your pharmacist regarding the use of digoxin.
		
		Check your potassium level constantly when taking digoxin. Low potassium level may put you at risk for digoxin toxicity and evidenced by severe nausea and vomiting and irregular heart beat.

Table 25h

HERBS AND PHYTOMEDICINAL AGENTS

Products: Common Name/Scientific Name	Description/Claimed Indications	Counseling Guidelines
NERVOUS SYSTEM DISORDERS: I. **Anxiety and Sleep Disorders** **Valerian** [*Valeriana officinalis*] 2-3 gm/day in divided doses 1-3 times/day. **Passion Flower** **Hops** **Catnip** **L-Tryptophan: Recalled! due to EMS** (see section on Sleep Aids) **Kava Kava**	Spasmolytic, mildly sedative, sleep aid.	Considered safe (see Sleep Aids). Avoid concurrent use of other central nervous system suppressents (barbiturates, sedative/hypnotics-benzodiazepines, opiates) and alcohol to avoid oversedation and hypotension.
II. **Depression** **St. John's Wort** [*Hypericum perforatum*] 2-4 gm of herb capsules or 0.2-1.0 mg hypericin.	Antidepressant for mild and moderate depression.	Generally safe. Photodermatitis may occur in light-skinned individuals. Avoid direct skin exposure to sunlight after ingesting the herb. Hypomania can also occur.
III. **Pain (General)** **Willow Bark** [*Salix alba*, etc.] 1-2 gm of finely powdered dried bark or 1-2 ml of tincture (1:5 25% ethanol) 3 times/day **Capsicum (e.g., Capsaicin in Zostrix)**	Inhibits prostaglandin synthesis in tissue and sensory nerves. Analgesic, anti-inflammatory, antipyretic, astringent activities. Indicated for rheumatic and arthritic conditions, common cold or influenza, mild headache, and gout.	St. John's Wort may cause increased antidepressant effect if taken with prescription antidepressants. Use with general anesthesia during surgery can cause unintended deepening of effect of anesthesia. Bupropion may cause increased antidepressant effect of St. John's Wort. Avoid concurrent use. Because of high tannin levels in therapeutic dose (0.75-5L of Willow bark tea), such a dose is ill-advised. **Consumers contemplating use of a crude Willow bark preparation as an analgesic or anti-inflammatory are best advised to use aspirin or other appropriate NSAIDs.**

HERBS & PHYTOMEDICINAL AGENTS

Products: Common Name/Scientific Name	Description/Claimed Indications	Counseling Guidelines
IV. Headache A. **Antimigraine Herbs** **Feverfew** [*Tanacetum parthenium*] 125 mg herb tablet or capsule daily.	Treat headaches, fevers, menstrual problems, and other painful maladies. Migraine headaches prophylaxis via inhibition of serotonin release.	GI discomfort and occasional mouth ulceration with fresh leaves may occur. Fever few may interact with blood thinners to cause bleeding. Avoid concurrent use.
B. **Caffeine-Containing Beverages Caffeine-Containing Plants:** [*Coffea arabica, Camellia sinensis, Cola nitida, Theobroma cacao, Paullinia cupana, Ilex paraguariensis*] 100-200 mg of caffeine/day. **Coffee** **Tea** **Kola (Cola)** **Cacao (Cocoa)** **Guarana** **Mate**	These herbs all contain caffeine (1,3,7-trimethylxanthine). Hence, are CNS stimulants, potentiate OTC analgesics by 40%, potentiate ergot alkaloids used for migraine headaches, and possess weak diuretic activity.	Caffeine-containing plants should be used with caution by persons with hypertension and related disorders. (See CNS Stimulants).
V. **Toothache** **Clove Oil** **Prickly Ash Bark**		
VI. **Sexual Impotence (Aphrodisiacs)** **Yohimbe (Yohimbine)** **Ginkgo**	Alpha-2-adrenergic blocking agent. Used in traditional medicine to treat angina, hypertension, and as halluicinogen. Aphrodisiac (stimulates sexual desire and performance). Used for treatment of impotence.	Yohimbine can cause severe hypotension, abdominal distress, and weakness. It should not be used in presence of renal and hepatic disease; should be taken under physician supervision. It can interact with all antihypertensives to cause severe hypotension, thereby attenuating the blood pressure-lowering effects of most antihypertensives. Avoid Yohimbine if you are currently receiving treatment for hypertension.

HERBS AND PHYTOMEDICINAL AGENTS

Products: Common Name/Scientific Name	Description/Claimed Indications	Counseling Guidelines
METABOLIC & ENDOCRINE DISORDERS:		
I. **Gynecological Disorders Black Cohosh** [*Cimicifuga racemosa*] 40-200 mg/day X 6 months.	Neurovisceral and psychic problems associated with menopause, premenstrual complaints, and dysmenorrhea.	GI discomfort, itching, rashes, have been reported. Contraindicated during pregnancy. Product contains alcohol.
Chaste Tree Berry [*Vitex agnus-castus*] Alcoholic extracts or tinctures contain: 20 mg of the crude fruit/day or 30-40 mg of the fruits in decoction/day X 166 days.	Menstrual problems (PMS), menstrual disorders due to primary or secondary corpus luteum insufficiency, mastalgia, menopausal symptoms, inadequate lactation.	
Evening Primrose Oil (EPO) [*Oenothera biennis*] or **Black Currant** [*Ribes nigrum*] or **Borage Seed** [*Borago officinalis*] 250 mg capsules. 600-6,000 mg/day for supplementaion; 1,000 mg 2 times daily for eczema. **Chaste Tree Berry Black Currant Oil Borage Seed Oil Raspberry Leaves** II. **Hyperthyroidism Bugle Weed** III. **Diabetes Mellitus: Petai? Malaysian Food!**	Precursor of prostaglandin E. For relief of symptoms of atopic eczema symptoms (e.g., itching). Supplementation in alcoholism and inflammation. GI disturbances may occur. Contraindicated during pregnancy and lactation. Preparation contains **60% alcohol (ethanol)**. Hence, may cause drowsiness. Consult your Pharmacist.	Generally safe. See section on Personal Hygiene. EPO may interact with phenothiazines (g.g.; chlorpromazine, thioridazine, fluphenazine) to increase incidence of seizures. EPO may also interact with anticonvulsants (e.g.; phenytoin, carbamazepine, valproic acid) to lower efficacy of the anticonvulsants. Avoid concurrent use.

HERBS AND PHYTOMEDICINAL AGENTS

Products: Common Name/Scientific Name	Description/Claimed Indications	Counseling Guidelines
ARTHRITIC &MUSCULOSKEL-ETAL DISORDERS: Disorders of the Skin, Mucous Membranes, and Gingiva. I. Dermatitis A. Tannin-Containing Herbs Witch Hazel or Hamamelis Water/Leaves [Hamamelis virginiana] Oak Bark English Walnut Leaves B. Other Herbal Products Chamomile Volatile Oil Evening Primrose Oil II. Contact Dermatitis Jewelweed III. Burns, Wounds, and Infections Aloe Vera Gel [Aloe vera] Arnica Calendula Comfrey Yogurt Tea Tree Oil (See Below)	Also see External Analgesics (Table 4) Contains 8-10% tannins which are responsible for the astringent activity of the herb. Also contains 14% **alcohol** for astringent effect. Therapeutically used as topical anti-inflammatory astringent and hemostyptics for minor skin injuries, hemorrhoids, and varicose veins. Anti-inflammatory, emollient (soothing properties). Enhances wound healing, hence, applied to first-degree burns and minor skin irritations.	Generally safe. Apply topically as necessary. Apply topically as necessary. The gel should not be confused with the yellow latex or juice occurring in specialized cells just below the leaf epidermis which is the source of the cathartic drug aloe. May cause skin irritation or allergies in sensitive individuals.

HERBS AND PHYTOMEDICINAL AGENTS

Products: Common Name/Scientific Name	Description/Claimed Indications	Counseling Guidelines
ARTHRITIC & MUSCULOSKEL-ETAL DISORDERS (continued): **Tea Tree Oi** [*Melaleuca alternifolia*]	Bacteriostatic and germicidal-used for treating boils, abscesses, sores, cuts, and abrasions, as well as wounds with pus discharge. Possible but not verified utility in the treatment of acne, arthritis, bruises, burns, cystitis, dermatitis, fungal infections, herpes, insect bites, muscular aches and pains, respiratory tract infections, sunburn, vaginal infections, varicose veins, and warts.	For topical application.

HERBS & PHYTOMEDICINAL AGENTS

Products: Common Name/Scientific Name	Description/Claimed Indications	Counseling Guidelines
IV. Lesions and Infections of the Oral Cavity and Throat A. CankerSores and Sore Throat **Goldenseal** [*Hydrastis canadensis*] 0.5-1 gm of the dried root or 2-4 ml of tincture (1:10, 60% ethanol) 3 times/day. **Rhatany** **Myrrh** **Guggul (Guggulu)** **Sage**	Antimicrobial, astringent, antihemorrhagic, in treatment of mucosal inflammation. A digestive tonic for the treatment of dyspepsia and gastritis.	Contraindicated in pregnancy.
B. Cold Sores **Melissa or Lemon balm** [*Melissa officinalis*] C. Dental Plaque 1. Significant Herbs **Bloodroot (Sanguinaria)** 2. Minor Herbs **Neem** **Mango** **Basil** **Tea** **Curry Leaves**	Calmative, spasmolytic, and carminative activity. May alleviate difficulty in falling asleep due to nervous conditions, and to treat functional GI symptoms. Antibacterial and antiviral activity against *Herpes simplex* type I (cold sores) and type II (genital herpes).	Apply topically as needed.

HERBS & PHYTOMEDICINAL AGENTS

Products: Common Name/Scientific Name	Description/Claimed Indications	Counseling Guidelines
ARTHRITIC & MUSCULOSKEL-ETAL DISORDERS: **V. Arthritis** **Willow Bark** **VI. Muscle Pain** **A. Rubefacients** **Volatile Mustard Oil** (Allyl Isothiocyanate) **Methyl Salicylate** **Turpentine Oil** **B. Refrigerants** **Menthol** **Camphor** **C. Other Counterirritants** **Capsicum (Capsaicin)**	Agents that induce redness and irritation. Agents that induce cooling sensation.	Also see section on External Analgesics

Table 25L

HERBS AND PHYTOMEDICINAL AGENTS

Products: Common Name/Scientific Name	Description/Claimed Indications	Counseling Guidelines
PERFORMANCE / ENDURANCE ENHANCERS ("Natural Stimulants), AND IMMUNE DEFICIENCIES:		
I. **Performance & Endurance Enhancers** **Ginseng** [*Panax ginseng*]: 1-2 gm daily.	Conflicting pharmacologic and clinical benefits: Radioprotective, antitumor, antiviral, metabolic, CNS, reproductive performance, lipid metabolism enhancement, antioxidant, cholesterol-lowering, and endocrinologic activities. Adaptogenic (facilitating resistance to various kinds of stress).	Generally considered safe if used appropriately. Ginseng products may contain up to **34% alcohol**. Besides the sedative and toxic effects of alcohol, it can also interact with many other medications. **Consult your pharmacist before using this product.**
Eleuthero or Siberian Ginseng [*Eleutherococcus senticosus*] 2-3 gm/day of the powdered or cut root in decoction. **Sarsaparilla** **Sassafras** **Ashwangandha** **Caffeine**	Adaptogenic activity in hyperthermia, elctroshock-induced convulsions, gastric ulcers, and x-ray irradiation. Increased metabolic efficiency in swimming -induced stress, improved conditioned response to stimuli, inhibition of conditioned avoidance response, antioxidant (free-radical scavenging), hypoglycemic, antiedema, anti-inflammatory, diuretic, gonadotropic, estrogenic, and antihypertensive activities.	Generally considered safe. Ginseng may increase the effects of estrogen, corticosteroids, digoxin, monoamine oxidase inhibitors, blood thinners (e.g.; warfarin, heparin) and oral hypoglycemics. Increased effect of blood thinners may cause bleeding. Avoid concurrent use.

HERBS & PHYTOMEDICINAL AGENTS

Products: Common Name/Scientific Name	Description/Claimed Indications	Counseling Guidelines
II. Communicable Diseases & Infection **Echinacea** [*Echinacea purpurea*] 6-9 ml/day [*Echinacea pallida*] 900 mg/day (tincture) [*Echinacea angustifolia*] 1 gm capsules, tablets, or tincture 3 times daily. **III. Cancer** **A. Significant Anticancer Herbs**	Non-specific immunostimulants, cold and flu prophylactics, treatment of *Candida albicans* infections. **Topical preparations** (ointments): for external treatment of hard-to-heal wounds, eczema, burns, psoriasis, herpes simplex, etc.	Do not use longer than 8 weeks; after that period, the immuno-stimulatory effects decline. Echinacea will antagonize the effects of immunosuppressants (e.g.; corticosteriods, cyclosporine, azathioprine)
Catharanthus [*Vinca rosea*]	Contains more than 70 alkaloids, including **Vinblastine** and **Vincristine**, which are extensively used in the treatment of a wide variety of malignant neoplasms.	Consult your physician or pharmacist for information regarding indications and adverse effects of the medications. Both alkaloids are prescription medications requiring administration by a qualified physician, pharmacist or nurse.

HERBS & PHYTOMEDICINAL AGENTS

Products: Common Name/Scientific Name	Description/Claimed Indications	Counseling Guidelines
Podophyllum	Alcoholic solution used as a topical treatment for certain papillomas (benign epithelial tumors). **Etoposide**, a semisynthetic derivative of one of the resin constituents, podophyllotoxin, has been developed. It is administered intravenously (IV) for the treatment of **testicular** and **ovarian germ cell cancers, lymphomas, small-cell lung cancers, and acute myelogenous and lymphoblastic leukemia.**	Consult your physician or pharmacist for information regarding these medications
Pacific Yew	Contains 0.01% of Paclitaxel (**Taxol**), a compound that has been found to be very useful when administered IV for the treatment of advanced ovarian cancer. Taxol shows considerable promise of becoming a useful chemotherapeutic agent in the treatment of ovarian cancer.	Consult your physician or pharmacist for information regarding this medication.
B. Unproven Anticancer Herbs		
Apricot		No proven value, hence Lack of therapeutic value
Pau d'Arco		Unproven value and cannot be recommended.
Mistletoe	Toxic plants. Potential antineoplastic effects when administered by injection	Their utility as nonspecific palliative therapy for malignant tumors remains unproven and is controversial.

Table 26a

SMOKING CESSATION PRODUCTS

Products/Description	Products/Description	Counseling Guidelines
CIGARETTE SMOKE: **Cigarette smoke contains:** a. 4,000 chemicals, 200 of them are poisons. b. 63 carcinogenic (cancer-causing) substances. c. Other toxic substances that are dangerous, although not necessarily cancer-causing. **Examples:** 1. **Ammonia:** A poisonous gas and common cleaning agent used in floor cleaners and detergents, and also for cleaning hypodermic equipment. 2. **Arsenic:** Was used as a rat poison. 3. **Carbon Monoxide (CO):** A colorless, odorless, poisonous gas present in automobile engine exhaust. CO can cause policythemia (increase in cell mass) via a response mechanism, requiring therapeutic phlebotomy, by binding to hemoglobin to form carboxyhemoglobin. The red blood cells thus loose their respiratory function.	4. **Naphthalene:** Used to make mothballs. 5. **Radioactive Compounds:** Used in nuclear weapons. 6. **DDT:** Used as an insecticide until 1971 when it was banned by the U.S. Food and Drug Administration because of its danger to the environment. Now its use is restricted. 7. **Formaldehyde:** An embalming fluid. Although there is not enough evidence that it acts as a carcinogen in humans, it certainly does in animals (Hoffman-AHF). 8. **Hydrogen Cyanide:** A gas proven to be extremely toxic to humans. The concentration of hydrogen cyanide in a cigarette is not enough to kill you, but at higher concentrations it is extremely toxic (Hoffman-AHF). It also is used as a rat and insect poison.	Before you light up a cigarette, ask yourself this question: **DO YOU KNOW WHAT YOU'RE SMOKING?** **You Can Quit!** Once you do quit, the health benefits start almost immediately; you will have more energy and feel less stressed (ALA). For information and useful tips to help you quit smoking, **contact:** 1. The American Lung Association (ALA): 1-800-586-4872 2. The American Cancer Society (ACS): 1-800-227-2345 3. Taking Care Health-Line: 1-800-933-4636, Code 2273 (CARE) 4. For your Free Smoking Cessation Kit, write to: **I'm Going To Kick Those Butts,** c/o Melanie Lutz, 8201 Greensboro Drive, Suite 500, McLean, VA 22102 {Offer limited to the first 1,000 individuals who respond (limit one per person)}

Table 26b

SMOKING CESSATION PRODUCTS

Products/Description	Product/Description	Counseling Guidelines
CIGARETTE SMOKE:	9. **Nicotine**: Used as an insecticide in agriculture and as a parasiticide in veterinary medicine. It is also a liver enzyme inducer which can cause decrease in blood concentration and hence faster elimination of many drug used concurrently. 10. **Benzene**: A poisonous gas. There also is significant evidence that benzene induces leukemia (Hoffman-AHF). 11. **Tar**: Inhibits mucociliary function in the upper respiratory tract resulting in predisposition to respiratory diseases (asthma & COPD).	Consequences of smoking include addiction, withdrawal symptoms, financial loss, heart disease, cancer, chronic obstructive pulmonary disease (COPD), asthma, pneumonia, teratogenicity, allergies, angina pectoris, cataracts, depression, glucose intolerance, Graves' disease, hypertension, peptic ulcer disaease, periodontal disease, peripheral vascular disease and death. Nicotine interacts with many medications resulting in lower blood levels and hence, efficacy of those drugs (analgesics, anticoagulants, cardiovascular agents - beta blockers, calcium channel blockers, furosemide, and other loop-type diuretics and thiazide diuretics, estrogens - estrogen replacements for postmenopausal women and oral contraceptives containing estrogens, H_2-antagonists - cimetidine, famotidine, nizatidine and ranitidine, insulin, psychotropics - barbiturates, benzodiazepines, phenothiazines and tricyclic antidepressants, theophylline, and vitamins. Consult your pharmacist if you are taking any of these medications.

SMOKING CESSATION PRODUCTS

Products	Description	Counseling Guidelines
I. **Nicotine Polacrilex Gum** [Nicorette] II. **Nicotine Transdermal Systems (NTS) 15 mg Patches** [Nicotrol, Nicoderm] III. **Nicotine Patch** [NicoDerm CQ] IV. **Nicotine Nasal Spray** 100 mg [Nicotrol NS] - (Rx - March 1996) V. **Nicotrol Inhaler -** (Rx - 1997) [Nicotine Inhahalation System (NIS)] VI. **Bupropion HCL** [Zyban] VII. **NicCheck I** **Note:** All are nicotine replacement dosage forms(i.e., substitute pharmacologically dosed nicotine for "smoked nicotine.")	**Nicotine Polacrilex** is available in **two package sizes**: a starter kit containing **108 Units** (about **2 weeks** of initial therapy) and a supplemental package containing **48 Units** (about **1 week** of therapy). Each package size is available in either **2 mg or 4 mg dose**. The **4 mg dosage** packages are targeted to those individuals who smoke more than 24 cigarettes per day. The package contains a **cassette tape** that provides instructions for use as well as a printed user's guide. NicCheck I is a 15-minute urine test that detects the presence of nicotine and its byproducts. It is a white strip that changes color when dipped in the urine of a smoker. The test will be useful for doctors and insurance companies checking patients who claim to have stopped smoking.	1. Consult your pharmacist or physician for directions for use of the nicotine products. 2. **Treatment lasts 12 weeks.** Then talk with your physician after this period. 3. Success of any nicotine reduction/cessation therapy depends on behavioral modification. 4. Stop smoking completely when you begin using this product. 5. Avoid consumption of acidic liquids while the dosing piece/gum is in the mouth. A basic pH is required for the nicotine to be properly released from the dosing piece into the saliva and then through the buccal mucosa. 6. Avoid exposing gum to extreme temperatures. 7. Keep this product out of the reach of children or pets (like all other medications). 8. Chewing the gum too quickly will result in an unpleasant taste caused by too much nicotine in the saliva. 9. Hiccups, nausea, an upset stomach, or a sore throat may result from improper use of the gum. 10. **One Nicotrol Patch should be applied daily for 6 weeks.** 11. Skin rash may occur at the site where the patch touches the skin. Rotating placement of the patch may alleviate this side effect.

ADVANTAGES OF NICOTROL, OVER OTHER NICOTINE PRODUCTS.

	NICOTROL	NICODERM CQ	NICORETTE
Proven effective to help smokers quit	✔	✔	✔
Simple one strength dose	✔		
No multiple step weaning process	✔		
Short 6-week therapy	✔		
Retail cost of total therapy	$175 per 6 weeks **$100 Savings!**	$280 per 10 weeks	$300-370 per 12 weeks

OTC Pharmaceutical Care: A Supplement to Drug Topics (PSI-100)
(Nicotine Transdermal System)

NICOTROL,
Is The Right Choice

FIRST-AID PRODUCTS AND MINOR WOUND CARE.

Products	Description	Counseling Guidelines

CATEGORY I FIRST-AID ANTISEPTICS
1. Alcohol (60-95%)
2. Benzalkonium chloride (0.1-0.13%)
3. Benzethonium chloride (0.1-0.2%)
4. Camphorated metacresol complex
5. Camphorated phenol complex
6. Combination of :
  eucalyptol (0.091%)
  menthol (0.042%)
  methylsalicylate (0.955%)
  and
  thymol (0.063%)
7. Hexylresorcinol (0.1%)
8. Hydrogen peroxide topical solution (H_2O_2) {USP}
 	
9. Iodine tincture {USP}
10. Iodine topical solution {USP}
11. Isopropyl alcohol (50-91.3%)
12. Methylbenzethonium chloride (0.13-0.5%), (creams, powders, solutions)
13. Phenol (0.5-1.5%)
14. Povidone-iodine complex (Betadine) (5-10%)
	H_2O_2 is an antimicrobial oxidizing agent and is the most widely used first-aid antiseptic. Enzymatic release of oxygen from H_2O_2 is followed by mechanical release (fizzing) of oxygen which has a cleansing effect on a wound.	These antiseptics are considered safe and effective (Category I).
		
		Alcohol (including isopropyl alcohol) may cause tissue irritation and skin dehydration at high concentration.
		
		Alcohol is also highly flammable and must be kept away from fire or flame.
		
		Use alcohol wash 3 times daily and cover with a sterile bandage after the washed area has dried.
		
		Bandaging should be discouraged after iodine application to avoid tissue irritation.
		
		Iodine absorption through the skin and mucous membranes can result in excess systemic iodine concentrations and can cause transient thyroid dysfunction, clinical hyperthyroidism, and thyroid hyperplasia.

FIRST-AID PRODUCTS AND MINOR WOUND CARE

Products	Description	Counseling Guidelines
FIRST-AID ANTIBIOTICS 1. Bacitracin+Neomycin+ Polymyxin (B+N+P) oint. Maximum Strength Neosporin, Neosporin ointment, Bactine First-Aid, Mycitracin Triple Antibiotic, N.B.P., Septa, Neomixin, Medi-Quick, Triple Antibiotic] 2. Bacitracin+Neomycin Cream [Neosporin] 3. Bacitracin+Polymyxin [Polysporin] ointment, powder, spray 4. Bacitracin 400-500 U/ gm ointment [Baciguent,..] 5. Neomycin 3.5 mg/gm [Myciguent, Various] 6. Tetracycline 3% ointment [Achromycin] 7. Chlortetracycline 3% ointment [Aueromycin]	Help **PREVENT infection** in minor cuts, wounds, scrapes, and burns.	Special caution should be taken when applying these preparations to denuded skin because the potential for systemic toxicity can increase. Prolonged use of these agents may result in secondary fungal infection. Consult a physician if healing does not occur within 5days. Allergic (hypersensitivity) reactions may be associated with these antibiotics. Discontinue use and consult a pharmacist or a physician if an allergy occurs. Apply 1-3 times daily and cover wound with a sterile bandage afterwards.

FIRST-AID PRODUCTS AND MINOR WOUND CARE

Products	Description/Use Indications	Counseling Guidelines
FIRST-AID WOUND MGT PRODUCTS **Transparent Adhesive Films:** 1. Polyurethane or Copolyester thin film [Acu-derm, Op-Site, Uniflex] 2. Nonadherent dressings [Adaptic, Telfa] 3. Alginates [Kaltostat, Sorbsan] 4. Exudate absorbers [Debrisan Beads, Hydragran] 5. Debriding agents 6. Gauze dressings (Nonocclusive fiber dressing with loose, open weave) 7. Hydrogels/Gels (Nonadherent, nonocclusive dressings [ElastoGel, Vigilon] 8. Composite/Island dressings [Nonadherent, adhesive at perimeter [Airstrip, Viasorb] 9. Foams (Polyurethane foam dressings) [APIGARD, LYOfoam] {Semipermeable, nonocclusive} 10. Hydrocolloids (Occlusive Wafer dressings) 11. Carbon-impregnated (Odor control) dressings [LYOfoam "C" Odor Absorbent Dressing] 12. Biosynthetics (Semipermeable dressings)[BioBrane II]	1. Semiocclusive dressing for stages I, II, shallow III wounds. Impermeable to fluids/bacteria. 2. Stages II, shallow III wounds, abrasions, lacerations. 3. Stages II, III, IV wounds. Hydrophilic dressings of Calcium-Na. 4. Stages II, III wounds. Hydrophilic dressings. 5. Stages II, III, some IV wounds. Dermal ulcers, 2nd and 3rd degree burns. 6. Stages II-IV wounds debridement, wound rehydration. 7. Stages II, III, some IV wounds. 8. Stages II, III, wounds. Impermeable to fluids/bacteria. 9. Stages II, shallow III, 1st and 2nd degree burns. Contraindicated for 3rd degree burns. 10. Stages I, II, and shallow III wounds. Hydrophilic and impermeable to fluids/bacteria. 11. For malodorous wounds. 12. Permeable to fluids/bacteria. **Note:** 1. Always clean the wound with mild soap and water or a mild wound cleanser that is not toxic to cells, avoiding antiseptic solutions unless they are extremely dilute. 2. Occlude the wound with a dressing that will keep the wound site moist and is an appropriate size and contour for the affected body part. 3. Avoid disrupting the dressing unnecessarily.	1. Will maintain a moist environment. Remove with caution to avoid reinjuring wound. 2. May require frequent dressing changes. 3. Will maintain moist a environment. Less frequent dressing changes required. 4. Maintain a moist environment. May be difficult to remove. Contraindicated with tunneling. 5. Need moist wound environment. May require frequent dressing changes. 6. Frequent dressing changes required. 7. Maintain moist environment. Most require frequent/daily dressing changes. 8. May cause periwound trauma on removal. 9. Less frequent dressing changes required. 10. Maintain a moist environment. May produce characteristic odor. 11. Control odor. Require appropriate seal or odor may escape. 12. Not for use on necrotic tissue. **Note:** 4. Use a mild analgesic to control pain. 5. Consult a physician if infection is suspected. Signs of infection include foul odors. Redness, swelling, and exudate are a normal part of healing. 6. Consult a physician if the wound occurred in dirty conditions and the patient's tetanus immunization status is uncertain.

PROBLEM-BASED LEARNING CASE SCENARIOS OR CASE STUDIES

CASE SCENARIO #1: SLEEP AID & CNS STIMULANT PRODUCTS	
Patient Complaint/History	**Clinical considerations/Strategies**
JC, a 28-year-old lawyer, presents to the pharmacist with a complaint of difficulty in sleeping for the past two nights. The patient, who is averaging only 5 hours of sleep instead of his usual 8, relates that once he falls asleep, he does not awake until the alarm goes off. He requests something to help him fall asleep. During further conversation, the patient reveals that he is giving a very important business presentation in 4 days; he seems to be "stressed out" about the presentation. He goes on to say that over the past week he has increased his caffeine consumption from the usual one cup of coffee with breakfast and lunch to two cups of coffee with each meal. JC has no known drug allergies and occasionally takes ibuprofen for muscle aches; he does not smoke and most weekends drinks only a few beers.	The following considerations/strategies are provided to aid the reader in a. determining whether treatment of the patient's condition with OTC medications is warranted, b. selecting the appropriate OTC medication, and c. developing a patient counseling strategy to ensure optimal therapeutic outcomes: 1. Identify factors that may be causing the sleep problems. 2. Identify principles of good sleep hygiene that may resolve the sleep problems. 3. Determine whether the patient has previously used any OTC sleep aid products. 4. Assess the value of therapy with an OTC sleep aid product; list the advantages and disadvantages of such therapy. 5. Identify key points about the OTC products (e.g., adverse effects, onset of action, duration of use) to discuss with the patient. 6. Identify symptoms whose occurrence would warrant the patient contacting a pharmacist or physician. 7. Develop a patient education/counseling strategy that will: - Explain the importance of good sleep hygiene; - Explain the advantages and disadvantages of any OTC medications used to treat the sleep problem. **DRUG CONSULT:**

PROBLEM-BASED LEARNING CASE SCENARIOS OR CASE STUDIES

CASE SCENARIO # 2: SLEEP AID & CNS STIMULANT PRODUCTS	
Patient Complaint/History	**Clinical Considerations/Strategies**
DK, a 25-year-old college student, presents to the pharmacist with a complaint of not being able to stay awake at night. Indicating the box of NoDoz in her hand, she asks if the medication will help her stay up at night. During further discussion, she reveals that she has several finals to take during the next week. DK also reveals that she was diagnosed as mildly hypertensive last year and has been taking Dyazide daily for the past year; she has a history of mitral valve prolapse. In addition to ibuprofen for occasional headaches, she takes the oral contraceptive Tri-Levlen 21 one tablet daily for 21 days, 7 days off. The patient, who is allergic to penicillin, reports that she does not smoke and drinks alcohol in moderation during social events. When asked about her diet and caffeine consumption, DK admits to drinking on average two cups of coffee with breakfast, two diet colas during the afternoon, and one glass of tea with dinner. She also eats a chocolate candy bar every afternoon.	The following considerations/strategies are provided to aid the reader in a. determining whether treatment of the patient's condition with OTC medications is warranted, b. selecting the appropriate OTC medication, and c. developing a patient counseling strategy to ensure optimal therapeutic outcomes: 1. Assess the appropriateness of the patient using NoDoz to help stay awake. 2. Assess the potential for drug-drug, drug-disease, and drug-dietary interactions if the patient were to take the NoDoz. 3. Determine whether the patient has used OTC stimulant products before. 4. Propose a response to the patient's original question: Will NoDoz help her stay awake at night? 5. Develop a patient education/counseling strategy that will: - Ensure that the patient understands the importance of the drug-drug, drug-disease, and drug-dietary interactions that might occur if NoDoz is taken; - Ensure that the patient understands what symptoms she may experience if she ingests too much caffeine and what she should do about them. **DRUG CONSULT:**

PROBLEM-BASED LEARNING CASE SCENARIOS OR CASE STUDIES

CASE SCENARIO #3: WEIGHT AND DIET CONTROL PRODUCTS	
Patient Complaint/History	**Clinical Considerations/Strategies**
PM, a 15-year-old local high school student, and her mother approach the pharmacy counter late one afternoon. The mother wants to ask the pharmacist, whom she considers her "neighborhood health expert," about the Dexatrim caplets she found in her daughter's back-pack. PM says that she takes the diet product "to get rid of this ugly fat." The mother wants to know whether the product is addictive or otherwise harmful. According to her mother, PM, who is 5'6" tall and weighs 128 lb, is in good health except for seasonal allergies associated with certain blooming plants. The package label identifies the diet product as Dexatrim Caffeine-Free Caplets; each caplet contains 75 mg of phenylpropanolamine in a sustained-release dosage form. PM reveals that she is also currently taking Dimetapp Allergy tablets "every so often"; the allergy medication was recommended by her pediatrician.	The following considerations/strategies are provided to aid the reader in a. determining whether treatment of the patient's condition with OTC medications is warranted, b. selecting the appropriate OTC medication, and c. developing a patient counseling strategy to ensure optimal therapeutic outcomes: 1. Ask the teenager why she thinks she needs to lose weight. 2. Assess the teenager's self-image and try to determine whether an underlying psychologic problem or other factors are behind the desire to lose weight. Be prepared to make appropriate referrals. 3. Determine the teenager's goals or desired effects from using the appetite suppressant (e.g., weight loss or stimulant effects). 4. Try to determine whether an underlying eating disorder is associated with the desire to lose weight. 5. Determine whether the teenager is eating a nutritionally balanced diet and whether she has tried to lose weight by modifying her intake of high-caloric and/or high-fat foods. 6. Explain to the teenager and her mother the proper role of OTC products in weight-loss programs as well as the limitations of such adjunctive products. 7. Determine whether the teenager is experiencing adverse effects consistent with CNS stimulant toxicity (e.g., jitteriness, irritability, insomnia, dizziness). 8. Explain to the teenager and her mother the potential consequences of duplicating the intake of phenylpropanolamine, which is an active ingredient in the allergy medication and the appetite suppressant. 9. Explain to the teenager and her mother the potential consequences of taking an OTC product without fully understanding the potential risks and benefits of the product. 10. Find out whether other girls at the patient's school are taking weight loss products; if so, find out what products they are taking. **DRUG CONSULT:**

PROBLEM-BASED LEARNING CASE SCENARIOS OR CASE STUDIES

CASE SCENARIO #4: INTERNAL ANALGESICS	
Patient Complaint/History JO, a 25-year-old female college student, presents to the pharmacist with complaints of a headache that she is unsure of how to treat. She has used ibuprofen, acetaminophen, or aspirin to relieve previous headaches; none of these medications caused adverse effects. When questioned about her symptoms, the patient describes a headache that may be related to sinus congestion; she feels pain in her forehead that intensifies in the morning. She has no other symptoms. JO has been taking decongestant/antihistamine (pseudoephedrine/chlorpheniramine) combination product, which has not relieved the sinus pain. To treat heartburn, she is also currently taking Pepcid AC 40 mg hs and antacids prn.	**Clinical Considerations/Strategies** The following considerations/strategies are provided to aid the reader in a. determining whether treatment of the patient's condition with OTC medications is warranted, b. selecting the appropriate OTC medication, and c. developing a patient counseling strategy to ensure optimal therapeutic outcomes: 1. Suggest an appropriate treatment regimen for the patient's headache. 2. Identify the precautions and adverse effects associated with the recommended OTC medication regimen. 3. Identify and assess medications you would not recommend to manage this patient's symptoms because of the presence of an ulcer. 4. Develop a patient/counseling strategy that will: - Ensure that the patient understands the appropriate use of the recommended OTC medication regimen; - Ensure that the patient understands when to contact a physician about her symptoms. **DRUG CONSULT:**

Table 28e

PROBLEM-BASED LEARNING CASE SCENARIOS OR CASE STUDIES

CASE SCENARIO #5: ANTACIDS	
Patient Complaint/History	**Clinical Considerations/Strategies**
RJ, a 46-year-old female, presents to the pharmacist with a complaint of fatigue. She goes on to explaun that for the past week she has been unable to perform her usual daily half-mile swim. Two weeks ago, she noticed a dull ache in her upper abdomen that was more pronounced at night and when she was hungry. The pain caused her to eat more often, increasing her weight by 4 lb. RJ's sister, who has a duodenal ulcer, recommended AlternaGEL for the stomach pain. Since taking the AlternaGEL, the patient has felt the stomach pain only at night.	The following considerations/strategies are provided to aid the reader in a. determining whether treatment of this patient's condition with OTC medications is warranted, b. selecting the appropriate OTC medication, and c. developing a patient counseling strategy to ensure optimal therapeutic outcomes:
Questions about the patient's lifestyle and dietary habits reveal that RJ smokes a pack of cigarettes a day, drinks a glass of wine with dinner every night, and drinks four cups of coffee during the day. When asked about the presence of other medical conditions, the patient explains that she was diagnosed with osteoarthritis of the right knee 5 years ago and that she has had occasional constipation for the past week. Her current medications include Motrin 400 mg q6h prn for pain; Fer-in-Sol 60 mg one capsule daily qAM; Centrum once daily qAM; Aristospan 10 mg intraarticular once a month; Ex-Lax 90 mg one tablet prn for constipation; and AlternaGEL 30 ml qid prn for pain.	1. Assess the possible causes of the fatigue and abdominal pain. 2. Determine the appropriateness of treating the abdominal pain with AlternaGEL. 3. Assess the effect of cigarette smoking, ethanol, and caffeine on this patient's condition. 4. Determine an appropriate response to the clinical situation. 5. Develop a patient education/counseling strategy that will: - Ensure that the patient understands the importance of discontinuing cigarette smoking and modifying her diet; - Ensure that the patient knows when to contact a health care provider. **DRUG CONSULT:**

PROBLEM-BASED LEARNING CASE SCENARIOS OR CASE STUDIES

CASE SCENARIO #6: LAXATIVES	
Patient Complaint/History	**Clinical Considerations/Strategies**
QA, a 66-year-old recently retired landscaper, walks up to pharmacy counter with two products in hand: Fleet Mineral OIL Enema and Kondremul. He explains that he is having a difficult time deciding betwen the two products. He also notes that he cannot remember being constipated since he became an adult. For occasional constipation during adolescence, his mother always gave him mineral oil. "It always seemed to work'"he says.	The following considerations/strategies are provided to aid the reader in a. determining whether treatment treatment of the patient's condition with OTC medications is warranted, b. selecting the appropriate OTC medication, and c. developing a patient counseling strategy to ensure optimal outcomes; 1. Determine whether this patient has constipation.
During questioning about his symptoms, the patient remarks that he should have come to the pharmacy 4 days ago; however, thinking that a good night's sleep would solve the problem, he picked up Benadryl capsules at a convenience store and has taken them for 3 nights. The patient reports that he is sleeping well but has had only one bowel movement in 9 days.	2. Assess the appropriateness of the active ingredient (mineral oil) in the patient-selected OTC products. 3. Assess the appropriateness of the dosage forms selected. 4. Assess the usefulness of dietary and lifestyle changes. 5. Consider the patient's age as a factor in recommending an OTC product.
After hearing the patient's description of his symptoms and attempted self-treatment, the pharmacist pulls up the patient's profile. The profile lists gouty arthritis, hypertension, and hyperlipidemia as chronic medical conditions for which the patient takes Capoten 25 mg bid; colchicine 0.6 mg bid; and Pravachol 10 mg bid, which was begun 3 weeks earlier. The patient has no known allergies.	6. Assess whether the patient's current drug therapy could play a role in the development of constipation. 7. Develop a patient education/counseling strategy that will: - Ensure that the patient understands the importance of the dietary and lifestyle modifications; - Ensure that the patient understands the proper use of the recommended OTC medications; - Ensure that the patient knows when to contact a health care provider. **DRUG CONSULT:**

PROBLEM-BASED LEARNING CASE SCENARIOS OR CASE STUDIES

CASE SCENARIO #7: COLD, COUGH, AND ALLERGY PRODUCTS	
Patient Complaint/History	**Clinical Considerations/Strategies**
YN, a 56-year-old female, presents to the pharmacist with symptoms of a severe viral infection of the upper respiratory tract. Her symptoms include profound nasal congestion, watery eyes, headache, malaise, and a dry, nonproductive cough. The patient reports that she feels warm; however, her oral temperature taken at 5:30 PM (about 30 minutes before arrival) was 98.9°F (37.5°C). YN also reveals that she has several chronic diseases, including hypertension, non-insulin-dependent diabetes, hyperlipidemia, and coronary artery disease. The patient's blood pressure has been in the range of 130-140 mmHg/80-85 mmHg for the last 6 months. Current prescription medications include hydrochlorothiazide 25 mg one tablet daily qAM for 6 years; Vasotec 10 mg one tablet daily qAM for 5 years; Micronase 10 mg one tablet daily with breakfast for 3 years; Zocor 20 mg one tablet daily qPM for last 8 months; and Nitrostat 0.4 mg one tablet (sublingual) prn for 1 month. YN selected the following OTC medications for the symptoms of her respiratory infection: Contac Maximum Strength 12-hour caplets; Tylenol Cold Medication; and Robitussin CF cough syrup. The patient has no known drug allergies.	The following considerations/strategies are provided to aid the reader in a. determining whether treatment of the patient's condition with OTC medications is warranted, b. selecting the appropriate OTC medication, and c. developing a patient counseling strategy to ensure optimal therapeutic outcomes: 1. Assess the appropriateness of the decongestant. 2. Assess the value of the cough syrup. 3. Assess the usefulness of an antihistamine in treating a viral infection of the upper respiratory tract (i.e., versus an allergy-mediated clinical situation). 4. Assess the ability of each patient-selected product to complicate the management of hypertension, diabetes, and coronary artery disease. 5. Determine which ingredients will have little positive impact on the patient's symptoms. 6. Propose an OTC medication regimen that is more targeted and focused to the symptoms associated with the respiratory infection. 7. Develop a patient education/counseling strategy that will: - Support/justify changes in the patient-selected OTC medication regimen; - Optimize proper use of the alternative OTC medication regimen recommended by the pharmacist. **DRUG CONSULT:**

PROBLEM-BASED LEARNING CASE SCENARIOS OR CASE STUDIES

CASE SCENARIO #8: HERBS AND PHYTOMEDICINAL PRODUCTS	
Patient Complaint/History	**Clinical Considerations/Strategies**
CP, an apparently health and obviously vigorous 64-year-old male, enters the consulting area and asks to speak privately with a pharmacist. The patient, who has patronized the pharmacy for several years, was diagnosed two years ago as having BPH for which his urologist prescribed Proscar 5 mg one tablet daily. His response to the medication has been excellent, but he now admits that the drug has greatly reduced his sexual potency. He also reveals that he plans to marry a 32-year-old woman; his first wife died 10 years ago. CP has read the *Physician's Desk Reference's* monograph on finasteride and is aware that the medication is probably the cause of his impotency. A friend who has no medical or pharmaceutical training advised him to quit taking finasteride and take saw palmetto standardized extract instead. CP asks whether this is a good idea. In addition to finasteride, he currently takes ascorbic acid (vitamin C) 250 mg one tablet daily and the standard OTC products for aches/pains and coughs/colds.	The following considerations/strategies are provided to aid the reader in a. determining whether treatment of the patient's condition with OTC medications is warranted, b. selecting the appropriate OTC medication, and c. developing a patient couseling strategy to ensure optimal therapeutic outcomes: 1. Assess the therapeutic use of saw palmetto as an alternative to finasteride. 2. Assess the appropriateness of recommending a dietary supplement as a substitute for a prescription medication. 3. Determine the best method for encouraging the patient's urologist to involved, remembering that the therapeutic use of botanicals is not usually taught in US medical schools. 4. Develop a patient education/counseling strategy that will: - Inform the patient of the need to consult his urologist before making any therapeutic decision; - Explain the effectiveness and limitations of saw palmetto standardized extract in treating BPH; - Aid the patient in selecting a specific botanical product and provide a suitable dosage regimen for the product (if the patient and his urologist collaborate and mutually approve a switch from Proscar to saw palmetto); - Explain the efficacy, side effect profile, and guidelines for the proper use of Proscar (if the patient and his urologist decide the switch is not appropriate). **DRUG CONSULT:**

PROBLEM-BASED LEARNING CASE SCENARIOS OR CASE STUDIES

CASE SCENARIO #9: SMOKING CESSATION PRODUCTS	
Patient Complaint/History	**Clinical Considerations/Strategies**
IJ, a 35-year-old female, presents to the pharmacist holding a carton of cigarettes and a 108-unit 4-mg package of Nicorette. Numerous prior attempts to help the patient stop smoking were unsuccessful. When questioned about the Nicorette, the patient indicates that she wishes to try to stop smoking "a little at a time" using this product. On separate occasions she previously tried a 24-hour and a 16-hour NTS without success. The patient admits that she just could not stop smoking, even when using the NTS. A review of IJ's patient profile reveals the following current prescriptions: propranolol 40 mg one tablet bid for hypertension (#60 filled monthly) and Nordette one tablet daily (#28 filled monthly). While filling the oral contraceptive prescription, the pharmacist notes the presence of tobacco flakes behind the tape covering the label on the container.	The following considerations/strategies are provided to aid the reader in a. determining whether treatment of the patient's condition with OTC drugs is warranted, b. selecting the appropriate OTC medication, and c. developing a patient counseling strategy to ensure optimal therapeutic outcomes: 1. Counsel the patient on potential interactions between smoking and her current medications. 2. Assess the willingness of the patient to stop smoking. 3. Determine why the NTS therapies might have failed. 4. Develop a pharmaceutical care plan for the patient's smoking cessation efforts and continue to educate and counsel the patient on smoking cessation options. 5. Contact the patient's physicians and explain the pharmaceutical care plan. DRUG CONSULT:

PROBLEM-BASED LEARNING CASE SCENARIOS OR CASE STUDIES

CASE SCENARIO #10: SMOKING CESSATION PRODUCTS	
Patient Complaint/History	**Clinical Considerations/Strategies**
SL, a 55-year-old male, calls the pharmacy to complain of a "racing heart beat." He reports that this effect first occurred when he began using nicotine polacrilex (40 4-mg dosing pieces a day) 10 days earlier and has continued throughout the therapy. He also complains of a sore throat that occurs after he drinks his customary six cups of coffee in the morning. When questioned about the presence of other symptoms, the patient reports that he has not suffered any withdrawal symptoms to date. He wants to stay off the cigarettes; however, the racing heart beat is frightening to him.	The following considerations/strategies are provided to aid the reader in a. determining whether treatment of the patient's condition with OTC drugs is warranted, b. selecting the appropriate OTC medication, and c. developing a patient counseling strategy to ensure optimal therapeutic outcomes: 1. Assess the probable cause of the patient's symptoms. 2. Contact the patient's primary physician to explain the symptoms as described by the patient. 3. Encourage the patient to come to the pharmacy for counseling.
A review of SL's patient profile reveals the following prescription medications: Theo-Dur 450 mg one tablet tid for asthma (#90 filled monthly); amoxicillin 500 mg one capsule tid for 10 days (filled 3 days earlier); Beconase AQ nasal spray 25 gm two sprays in each nostril bid (filled monthly); and Claritin-D one tablet bid for 10 days (#20 filled 3 days earlier).	4. Review with the patient the proper dosing technique for administraion of the nicotine polacrilex therapy. 5. Suggest a dosage regimen and caution the patient about concurrent consumption of acidic beverages. 6. Develop a pharmaceutical care plan for the patient's smoking cessation program. 7. Work with the physician and the patient to determine a potential revision in the theophylline dosage. **DRUG CONSULT:**

Adapted from reference 2

SAMPLE CASE SCENARIO: Patient Counseling Challenge.

Pharmacist: "Hi, I'm Roberta Armstrong. How may I help you today?"

Patient: "Well, I just was out to the store and I had some questions. They said I could come and see you."

Pharmacist: "Please have a seat."

Patient: "Thank you. I tell you, last night I had some spicy food for dinner and when I went to bed, I lay down, but I didn't get much sleep and here we are like 14 hours later and I'm still feeling this heartburn, and it's not going away. So I was going to ask, is there some kind of preparartion I can get from you?"

Pharmacist: "Okay. First I need to ask you a series of questions. Is that okay, in order to determine the best possible treatment?"

Patient: "Sure."

Pharmacist: "Okay, who has the problem? You definitely have the problem."

Patient: "It's me. Yeah."

Pharmacist: "Okay. And when did you see a physician the last time and why?"

Patient: "Oh, I had my annual check-up about six-eight months ago. Just an annual check-up."

Pharmacist: "You've never seen a physician for this particular condition?"

Patient: "No."

Pharmacist: "So, how long have you had this problem?"

Patient: "Well, this is going back quite a while now. I guess a few years."

Pharmacist: "Okay. What other medications are you taking, both prescription and over-the-counter?"

Patient: "Well, I'm not taking any prescription drugs and over-the-counter, you know, maybe take some aspirins. Nothing recently."

Pharmacist: "Do you see any indication of upset stomach after taking aspirin?"

Patient: "No."

Pharmacist: "What medications have you tried for this particular condition?"

Patient: "My wife gave me some of this white liquid and some chalky tablets last night but it didn't do the trick."

SAMPLE CASE SCENARIO: Patient Counseling Challenge.

Pharmacist:
"Okay. First I need to ask you a series of questions. Is that okay, in order to determine the best possible treatment?"

Pharmacist: "Have you tried any lifestyle changes like elevating your bed six to eight inches at the head?"

Patient: "No, I haven't."

Pharmacist: "How about loosening tight clothing or, if you're a smoker, quit smoking, or losing weight?"

Patient: "No. Well, I'm not a smoker. I haven't tried the others. Maybe I'll give them a try."

Pharmacist: "Okay. When you have the pain, does it elevate up into the chest or down into the abdomen?"

Patient: "It seems to go just like right in here."

Pharmacist: "Okay, not down..."

Patient: "Yeah, like a burning feeling."

Pharmacist: "Okay. Do you have any coughing with it?"

Patient: "No."

Pharmacist: "Pain or difficulty in swallowing?"

Patient: "No."

Pharmacist: "Okay. Do you have any change in your stool? Black tar or any bright blood, or vomiting, any..."

Patient: "Gee, no. I don't have any of those problems."

Pharmacist: "Nothing. Weight loss?"

Patient: "No."

Pharmacist: "Okay. What I'm going to recommend is Pepcid AC for acid control. The generic name of the it is famotidine. As far as the dosage, it seems like you need to take it one hour before you have the problem, such as with spicy food, or you can take one after you have the problem. The dosage is one tablet up to two times a day but not more than two tablets in 24 hours. And the important thing to remember is to not increase the dosage. If you have to take it consecutively for two weeks, then it's important to check with a physician. Or if you see any symptoms I described, like the blood in the stool, black tarry stool, or pain or difficulty in swallowing, it's important to check with your physician. If the Pepcid AC doesn't help in a few days, make sure to call your doctor."

Source: U.S. Pharmacist 1996;21(6):122-123.

SAMPLE OTC NAPLEX REVIEW EXAMINATION

DIRECTIONS: Each question below contains five (5) suggested answers.
Choose the **ONE BEST** response to each question.

1. According to the FDA categorization, the following OTC drug ingredients are recognized as safe and effective for the claimed therapeutic indication:
   a. Class II
   b. Category III
   c. Category I
   d. Third Class
   e. None of these

2. Once a drug is approved by the FDA, the patent of the brand name by the manufacturer is good for how long?
   a. 5 years
   b. 10 years
   c. 17 years
   d. An indefinite period
   e. The life of the manufacturer

3. Pepcid **AC** and Tagamet **HB** are recent Rx-to-OTC products which belong to the following pharmacological class:
   a. Non-steroidal antiinflammatory agents
   b. Antifungal drugs
   c. Antihypertensive agents
   d. H_2-antagonists
   e. Antiviral drugs

4. The following OTC analgesic/antipyretic agent may be considered safest in pregnancy:
   a. Tylenol®
   b. Anacin®
   c. Motrin®
   d. Aleve®
   e. Ecotrin®

5. Which of the following laxatives would you recommend for a pregnant women who complains of occasional constipation?
   a. Metamucil®
   b. Bisacodyl
   c. Phenolphthalein

| | d. | Fleet's enema |
| | e. | Cascara sagrada |

6. Antihistamines are used in OTC cold preparations for their:
   - a. Histamine-blocking action
   - b. Anticholinergic effects
   - c. Vasodilating effects
   - d. Microsomal enzyme-inducing effects
   - e. Sedating effects

7. Active ingredients of OTC cold and allergy products containing guaifenesin, pseudoephedrine and dextromethorphan would have a/an:
   - a. Antihistamine, decongestant, and antitussive
   - b. Expectorant, decongestant, and antitussive
   - c. Demulcent, antihistamine, and antitussive
   - d. Expectorant, demulcent, and antitussive
   - e. Antitussive, decongestant, and demulcent

8. Which of the following OTC cold medications contains the ingredients pseudoephedrine and triprolidine?
   - a. Actifed®
   - b. Sudafed®
   - c. Drixoral®
   - d. Dristan®
   - e. Dimetapp®

9. The following OTC expectorant contains alkaloids emetine and cephaeline which are highly toxic:
   - a. Terpin hydrate
   - b. Ipecac
   - c. Guaifenesin
   - d. Ammonium chloride
   - e. Noscapine

10. Which of the following OTC cold products will antagonize histamine release from mast cells?
   - a. Chlortrimeton
   - b. Sudafed
   - c. Phenylephrine
   - d. Pseudoephedrine
   - e. Benzonatate

11. The following class of antihistamines is the least sedating for your client's rhinorrhea:
   - a. Ethanolamines
   - b. Ethylenediamines
   - c. Alkylamines

d.   B and C are equally sedating

e.   All are equally sedating

12.   Vegetarians are considered a particularly high risk group for developing:

a.   Xerosis

b.   Pernicious Anemia

c.   Skin Cancer

d.   Cataracts

e.   Cirrhosis

13.   Which of the following drugs has been shown to cause folic acid deficiency?

a.   Amoxicillin

b.   Allopurinol

c.   Leucovorin

d.   Trimethoprim

e.   Warfarin

14.   Kendrix Harry enters your pharmacy complaining of decreased hearing , pain and ringing in the ear. You look in his ear and find that there are no visible signs of redness or swelling. Your recommendation to Mr. Harry could include:

a.   Carbamide Peroxide 6.5% drops

b.   Diluted Hydrogen Peroxide

c.   Irrigation with a mixture of 20-30% alcohol and water

d.   All of the above

e.   None of the above

15.   Common OTC decongestants used for topical application to the nasal passages include:

I.   Phenylephrine HCl and naphazoline

II.   Oxymetazoline HCl and xylometazoline HCl

III.   Phenylpropanolamine HCl and pseudoephedrine sulfate

a.   I only

b.   III only

c.   I and II only

d.   II and III only

e.   I, II and III

16.   Which of the following decongestant(s) is/are associated with rebound nasal congestion from chronic use?

I.   Xylometazoline

II.   Oxymetazoline

III.   Phenylephrine

a.   I only

b.   III only

c.   I and II only

d.   II and III only
e.   I, II and III

17.   Common errors associated with the use of Metered-Dose Inhalers include:
    I.   inhaling completely and then actuating the device
    II.   actuating the device and holding breath without inhaling
    III.   waiting 1-2 minutes between puffs

    a.   I only
    b.   III only
    c.   I and II
    d.   II and III
    e.   I, II, and III

18.   When dispensing beclomethasone dipropionate inhalers (Vanceril®), you must always advise the patients to rinse the mouth after administration because of the following reason(s):
    I.   Corticosteroids may predispose individuals to oral yeast infection
    II.   Corticosteroids stimulate appetite and may cause the patient to gain weight
    III.   Beclomethasone is an anticoagulant and may cause bleeding of the gums

    a.   I only
    b.   III only
    c.   I and II
    d.   II and III
    e.   I, II, and III

19.   Which of the following statements is/are true?
    I.   Retinoids are Vit. A
    II.   Calciferols are Vit. C
    III.   Tocopherols are Vit. D

    a.   I only
    b.   III only
    c.   I and II only
    d.   II and III only
    e.   I, II and III are correct

20.   Vitamin C deficiency may be associated with:
    I.   Deterioration of the skin and connective tissues
    II.   Degeneration of the teeth and gums

III. Abnormal bleeding in the skin
a. I only
b. III only
c. I and II only
d   II and III only
e. I, II and III

21. Which of the following medications is NOT available OTC?
a. Elase
b. Basaljel
c. Docusate
d. Humulin N
e. Ensure Plus

22. Miconazole is indicated to treat infections caused by which of the following?
a. Candida albicans
b. Neisseria gonorrhoeae
c. Chlamydaia trachomatis
d. Staphylococcus aureus
e. Streptococcus pyogenes

23. Benadryl® possesses all of the following properties EXCEPT:
a. antihistaminic
b. antipruritic
c. antikeratolytic
d. antitussive
e. anticholinergic

24. The initial milk from the breast is referred to as:
a. Casein
b. Chymotrypsin
c. Colostrum
d. Alimentum
e. Nutramigen

25. Ms. Ecker needs no prescription to purchase which of the following?
I.   Fero-Folic-500
II. Miconazole
III. Colace

a. I only
b. III only
c. I and II only
d. II and III only
e. I, II, and III

26. Mr. Jackson asks the pharmacist to recommend a hay fever remedy. The product **LEAST** likely to exacerbate Mr. Jackson's Parkinson's disease and hypertension is:

    a.   Contac.
    b.   Comtrex.
    c.   Dristan Advanced Formula.
    d.   Sinutab Maximum Strength.
    e.   Tavist-1

27. A patient who has an enlarged prostate should be advised **NOT** to take:

    I.   antihistamines.
    II.   sympathomimetics.
    III.   salicylates.

    a.   I only
    b.   III only
    c.   I and II only
    d.   II and III only
    e.   I, II, and III

28. Which of the following is the active ingredient in Metamucil® ?

    a.   an anthraquinone glycoside.
    b.   a hydrocolloid.
    c.   a hyperosmotic polymer.
    d.   a cellulose derivative.
    e.   a surfactant.

29. The same active ingredient is found in Metamucil® and in which of the following?

    I.   Effer-syllium.
    II.   Fiberall.
    III.   Citrucel.

    a.   I only
    b.   III only
    c.   I and II only
    d.   II and III only
    e.   I, II, and III

30. The most appropriate agent to recommend as treatment of crab lice is:

    a.   NP-27.
    b.   A-200 pyrinate.
    c.   Absorbine Jr.
    d.   Cruex.
    e.   Komed.

31.   **EXCEDRIN** contains which of the following combinations of ingredients?
     a.   ASA / APAP / Caffeine
     b.   ASA / Phenyltoloxamine
     c.   ASA / Caffeine
     d.   APAP / Caffeine
     e.   none of the above

32.   Which statement (s) is/are **TRUE** ?
     I.   Acetaminophen is very safe when taken correctly
     II.   Acetaminophen's antiplatelet effect is reversible
     III.   Acetaminophen is an antiinflammatory agent

     a.   I only
     b.   III only
     c.   I and II
     d.   II and III
     e.   I, II, and III

33.   Docusate is classified pharmacologically as:
     a.   a fecal softener.
     b.   a bulk laxative.
     c.   a hyperosmolar agent.
     d.   a stimulant cathartic.
     e.   an irritant laxative.

34.   Which method of testing for glucose does **NOT** use glucose oxidase?
     a.   Tes-tape
     b.   Clinitest
     c.   Diastix
     d.   Chemstrip uG
     e.   Clinistix

35.   What contraceptive is most effective in preventing venereal disease?
     a.   Vaginal sponge
     b.   Spermicidal foam
     c.   Diaphragm
     d.   Condom
     e.   IUD

36.   Which of the following statements is/are **TRUE** regarding the One Touch and Accu-Chek EZ blood glucose monitors?
     I.   Both give results in 45 seconds.
     II.   Wiping is required for both
     III.   The Accu-Chek EZ blood glucose range is up to 600mg/dl and One Touch is up to 800mg/dl.

a. I only
b. III only
c. I and II
d. II and III
e. I, II, and III

37. A patient asks for a product to detect blood in the stool. The pharmacist should appropriately recommend:
a. First Response.
b. One Touch II.
c. AccuCheck.
d. EZ-Detect.
e. Tracer II.

38. How is Human insulin manufactured ?
a. high performance liquid chromatography
b. recombinant DNA process using E. Coli
c. semisynthetic cattle insulin
d. harvest from apes
e. chemical manipulation bovine insulin

39. _____ are used to treat certain minor bacterial infections (i.e. Staphylococcal blepharitis)
I. Astringents
II. Antipruritics
III. Anti-microbials

a. I only
b. III only
c. I and II only
d. II and III only
e. I, II, and III

40. The treatment for chlamydial conjunctivitis is_____.
I. Ocular decongestants
II. Artificial tear preparations
III. An Rx antibiotic

a. I only
b. III only
c. I and II only
d. II and III only
e. I, II, and III

41. The imidazole(s) with the greatest propensity for rebound congestion include:
   I.   Oxymetazoline
   II. Naphazoline
   III. Tetrahydrozoline

   a. I only
   b. III only
   c. I and II only
   d. II and III only
   e. I, II, and III

42. Hard lens maintenance involves several important steps. They are:
   I.   Cleaning
   II. Soaking
   III. Wetting

   a. I only
   b. III only
   c. I and II only
   d. II and III only
   e. I, II, and III

43. Increased concentrations of prostaglandins have been implicated as an etiological factor in:
   I.   Amenorrhea
   II. Lactation
   III. Dysmenorrhea

   a. I only
   b. III only
   c. I and II
   d. II and III
   e. I, II and III

44. The mechanism of action of nonsteroidal anti-inflammatory drugs is:
   I.   inhibiting prostaglandin synthesis
   II. inhibiting the cough reflex center of the medulla oblongata
   III. inhibiting peptide synthesis

   a. I only
   b. III only
   c. I and II
   d. II and III
   e. I, II and III

45. Intermenstrual bleeding is believed to be caused by a temporary decrease in:
    I.   norgestrel
    II. progestin
    III. estrogen

    a. I only
    b. III only
    c. I and II
    d. II and III
    e. I, II and III

46. To prevent symptoms of milk intolerance, Mr. Gibberman coulld appropriately ingest dairy products with the following OTC product:
    a. Lacril.
    b. LactAid.
    c. lactulose.
    e. lactic acid.

47. Mitrolan can be classified as which type of laxative?
    a. Anthraquinone
    b. Hyperosmotic
    c. Stimulant
    d. Saline
    e. Bulk

48. A cardiac patient is instructed to take a combination fecal softener/stimulant for constipation. The pharmacist should appropriately recommend:
    a. Milk of magnesia.
    b. Colace.
    c. Senokot.
    d. Doxidan.
    e. Ex-Lax.

49. Vitamin B6 is usually recommended to patients to prevent peripheral neuritis which is associated with the use of:
    a. Isoniazid
    b. Rifampin
    c. Ethambutol
    d. Pyrazinamide
    e. Cycloserine

50. When dispensing Ansaid® 100 mg bid, the pharmacist should caution against the concomitant use of:
    I.   aspirin.
    II. alcohol.
    III. antacids.

a. I only
b. III only
c. I and II
d. II and III
e. I, II and III

51. Evening Primrose Oil (can be used in premenstrual syndrome) contains gamma linoleic acid which is a precursor of prostaglandin _____.
   I. E1
   II. PGE2
   III. PGI2

   a. I only
   b. III only
   c. I and II
   d. II and III
   e. I, II and III

52. This fat-soluble vitamin has been evaluated in the treatment of PMS.
   I. vitamin A
   II. vitamin K
   III. vitamin E

   a. I only
   b. III only
   c. I and II
   d. II and III
   e. I, II and III

53. The following medications may predispose a woman to yeast infections:
   I. immunosuppressants
   II. chemotherapeutic agents
   III. non-steroidal anti-inflammatory agents

   a. I only
   b. III only
   c. I and II
   d. II and III
   e. I, II and III

54. Patients who are _____ often experience more yeast infections than normal patients.
   I. hypertensive
   II. immunosuppressed
   III. diabetic

a. I only
b. III only
c. I and II
d. II and III
e. I, II and III

55. What OTC product is indicated for either diarrhea or constipation?
    a. Donnagel
    b. Mitrolan
    c. Kaopectate
    d. Senokot
    e. Colace

56. Factor(s) to consider in choosing a method of birth control include:
    I. safety profile
    II. efficacy profile
    III. patient acceptance

    a. I only
    b. III only
    c. I and II
    d. II and III
    e. I, II and III

57. The following is/are classified as spermicidal agents:
    I. Menfegol
    II. Octoxynol 9
    III. Nonoxynol 2000

    a. I only
    b. III only
    c. I and II
    d. II and III
    e. I, II and III

58. Spermicides are available in which of the following dosage forms?
    I. jelly
    II. cream
    III. suppository

    a. I only
    b. III only
    c. I and II
    d. II and III
    e. I, II and III

59. Latex male condoms have been shown to demonstrate efficacy against:
    I.   Human Immunodeficiency Virus (HIV)
    II. Sexually Transmitted Diseases (STDs)
    III. Chlamydia

    a. I only
    b. III only
    c. I and II
    d. II and III
    e. I, II and III

60. Common causes of failure with male condoms include:
    I.   the use of oil-based lubricants
    II. improper use
    III. air is not squeezed out of the tip of the condom

    a. I only
    b. III only
    c. I and II
    d. II and III
    e. I, II and III

61. Feminine hygiene products include which of the following?
    I.   vaginal cleansing products
    II. feminine napkins and tampons
    III. personal lubricants

    a. I only
    b. III only
    c. I and II
    d. II and III
    e. I, II and III

62. A number of products are available to alleviate minor vaginal discomfort of itching. Most of these products contain hydrocortisone in a concentration of:
    I.   0.5% - 1%
    II. 1% - 2%
    III. 0.5% - 2%

    a. I only
    b. III only
    c. I and II
    d. II and III
    e. I, II and III

63. Thiamine is indicated for which of the following conditions?
   a. Wernicke-Korsakoff syndrome.
   b. Stevens-Johnson syndrome.
   c. hepatic encephalopathy.
   d. macrocytic anemia.
   e. delirium tremens.

64. A patient who has been regularly taking Tagamet® for the treatment of an active peptic ulcer requests an OTC analgesic. The pharmacist can appropriately recommend:
   a. Nuprin®.
   b. Anacin®.
   c. Tylenol®.
   d. Bufferin®.
   e. Ascriptin®.

65. Appropriate OTC preparations for athlete's foot include all of the following, **EXCEPT**:
   a. NP-27.
   b. Aftate.
   c. Desenex.
   d. Tinactin.
   e. Mycitracin.

66. The following agents are commonly found in dentifrices. Which agent facilitates the removal of plaque?
   a. sodium fluoride
   b. zinc chloride
   c. silica
   d. sodium bicarbonate
   e. both a and b

67. Which of the following dentifrices would NOT be a good choice in a person with sensitive teeth?
   I. Pearl Drops Toothpolish with Fluoride
   II. Colgate Tartar Control Paste
   III. Crest Winterfresh Gel with Peroxide and Baking Soda RDA

   a. I only
   b. III only
   c. I and II only
   d. II and III only
   e. I, II, and III

68. The following ethanolamine antihistamine is the only FDA-approved agent for the

treatment of short-term insomnia

    I.   Chlortrimeton®
    II.   Unisom®
    III.   Nytol®

    a.   I only
    b.   III only
    c.   I and II
    d.   II and III
    e.   I, II, and III

69.   Diphenhydramine HCL has all of the following properties, **EXCEPT**:

    a.   antiemetic
    b.   antitussive
    c.   emetic
    d.   antihistaminic
    e.   sedative/hypnotic

70.   The following potent methylxanthine derivative is the only FDA-approved OTC stimulant for occasional use.

    I.   ephedrine sulfate
    II.   ephedrine sulfate + theophylline + phenobarbital combination product
    III.   Vivarin®

    a.   I only
    b.   III only
    c.   I and II
    d.   II and III
    e.   I, II and III

71.   Which of the following OTC anorexiants (anorectics) works by causing alteration of taste sensation and consequently loss of appetite?

    a.   MS Dexatrim®
    b.   Acutrim 16 Hour®
    c.   Slim-Mint®
    d.   MS Dex-A-Diet®
    e.   Acutrim Late Day®

72.   The most common adverse effect associated with magnesium-containing antacids is:

    a.   fever
    b.   constipation
    c.   diarrhea
    d.   tachycardia

e.   urinary retention

73.   The most commonly reported untoward effect of aluminum-containing antacids is:
        a.   constipation
        b.   diarrhea
        c.   dry mouth
        d.   neuroleptic malignant syndrome

74.   Maalox and Mylanta usually contain an antiflatulent agent called:
        a.   alginic acid
        b.   attapulgite
        c.   simethicone
        d.   milk of magnesia
        e.   none of the above

75.   To avoid chelation/complexation (interaction) between antacids and
tetracycline, you must advise your patients as follows:
        a.   separate doses by 1-2 hours
        b.   take with dairy products
        c.   take with food
        d.   take both drugs at the same time
        e.   none of the above

76.   Alka-Seltzer® contains which of the following?
        a.   sodium carbonate
        b.   sodium bicarbonate
        c.   calcium carbonate
        d.   magnesium citrate
        e.   aluminum oxide

77.   Cimetidine can interact with theophylline to cause which of the following?
        I.   decrease theophylline levels
        II.   no effect on theophylline levels
        III.   increase theophylline levels

        a.   I only
        b.   III only
        c.   I and II
        d.   II and III
        e.   I, II and III

78.   The following antidiarrheal agent works by adsorbing the diarrhea-causing agents
in the GI tract:
        a.   Rheaban
        b.   Imodium

    c.   Imodium AD

    d.   Belladonna alkalloids

    e.   atropine

79.   Which of the following stool softeners is known to cause severe GI irritation due to the presence of casanthranol?

    a.   Colace

    b.   Pericolace

    c.   Docusate calcium

    d.   all of above

    e.   none of the above

80.   The following laxative is recommended for a patient with a history of hypertension and/or congestive heart failure.

    I.   docusate sodium

    II.   docusate sodium with casanthranol

    III.   docusate calcium

    a.   I only

    b.   III only

    c.   I and II

    d.   II and III

    e.   I, II and III

81.   Enemas are designed for what route of administration?

    a.   oral

    b.   rectal

    c.   parenteral

    d.   intrathecal

    e.   epidural

82.   All of the following are hemorrhoidal preparations **EXCEPT**:

    a.   Benzocaine

    b.   Pramoxine HCL

    c.   Preparation H

    d.   Anusol-HC

    e.   Emetrol

83.   The expectorant **terpin hydrate** has which of the following properties?

    I.   It acts by bronchial stimulation

    II.   It decreases mucus production

    III.   It decreases mucus viscosity

    a.   I only

    b.   III only

c. I and II only
d. II and III only
e. I, II and III

84. Ingredients with antitussive action that may be found in OTC cough preparations include:
I. Dextromethorphan
II. Diphenhydramine
III. Hydrocodone

a. I only
b. III only
c. I and II only
d. II and III only
e. I, II and III

85. Dextromethorphan may be equipotent to codeine but has the following distinguishing characteristics:
I. Non-analgesic activity
II. No addictive potential
III. It is a narcotic

a. I only
b. III only
c. I and II only
d. II and III only
e. I, II and III

86. Which of the following OTC cold products possesses sedative as well as anticholinergic properties?
I. Diphenhydramine
II. Noscapine
III. Phenylephrine

a. I only
b. III only
c. I and II only
d. II and III only
e. I, II and III

87. Codeine SO_4 (OTC in Puerto Rico and other countries) is known to cause which of the following adverse effects?
I. Drowsiness
II. Constipation
III. Addiction

a. I only
b. III only
c. I and II only
d. II and III only
e. I, II and III

88. Goals of proper use of Metered-Dose inhalers include which of the following?
     I.   minimize amount of drug lost in the upper airways
     II.   maximize deposition of drug by gravitational force into the lower airways
     III.   maximize amount of drug lost in the upper airways

     a. I only
     b. III only
     c. I and II
     d. II and III
     e. I, II, and III

89. The following blood pressure instrument utilizes a microphone which is placed directly over the patient's artery for blood sounds detection:
     I.   mercury sphygmomanometer
     II.   aneroid sphygmomanometer
     III.   electronic blood pressure meter

     a. I only
     b. III only
     c. I and II
     d. II and III
     e. I, II, and III

90. In the Fecal Occult Blood Test, the Hgb peroxidase enzyme is responsible for the following activity:
     I.   reduction of the test reagent
     II.   conjugation of the test reagent
     III.   oxidation of the test reagent

     a. I only
     b. III only
     c. I and II
     d. II and III
     e. I, II, and III

91. The following solutions are used to remove blood stains from hypodermic equipment:

130

I.   0.9% HNO_3
II.   10% HNO_3
III.   concentrated ammonia (NH_3)

a.   I only
b.   III only
c.   I and II
d.   II and III
e.   I, II, and III

92.   Humidifiers work by which of the following mechanisms?
       I.   reducing the viscosity of the tenacious mucus in the respiratory airway
       II.   providing reservoir for drug between actuation and inhalation
       III.   measuring the amount of moisture in the atmosphere

a.   I only
b.   III only
c.   I and II
d.   II and III
e.   I, II, and III

93.   In selecting a needle for your patient, the following considerations are necessary:
       I.   fluidity of liquid to be administered
       II.   safety and comfort of patient
       III.   desired depth of penetration

a.   I only
b.   III only
c.   I and II
d.   II and III
e.   I, II, and III

94.   Advantages of ambulatory blood pressure monitoring include the following:
       I.   evaluation of effectiveness of high blood pressure therapy
       II.   avoidance of "white Coat" phenomenon
       III.   early detection of elevated blood pressure

a.   I only
b.   III only
c.   I and II
d.   II and III
e.   I, II, and III

95.   Which of the following topical anesthetics has the highest incidence of sensitiza-

tion?

    a.   lidocaine
    b.   benzocaine
    c.   pramoxine
    d.   dibucaine
    e.   a and b are correct

96.   Which of the following properties do/does zinc oxide possess?
    I.   protectant
    II.   astringent
    III.   sunblock

    a.   I only
    b.   III only
    c.   I and II only
    d.   II and III only
    e.   I, II, and III

97.   Which of the following properties of hydrocortisone are beneficial in the management of dermatitis?
    I.   Treats and relieves the dermatitis
    II.   Relieves itching
    III.   Exacerbates infections

    a.   I only
    b.   III only
    c.   I and II only
    d.   II and III only
    e.   I, II, and III

98.   What is the active ingredient in Head and Shoulders dandruff shampoo?
    a.   salicylic acid
    b.   sulfur
    c.   selenium sulfide
    d.   zinc pyrithione
    e.   coal tar

99.   Which of the following properties does camphor possess?
    I.   antiseptic
    II.   counterirritant
    III.   rubefacient

    a.   I only
    b.   III only
    c.   I and II only

    d.   II and III only
    e.   I, II, and III

100.   Which category of agents contain(s) salicylate derivatives as an active ingredient?

    I.   sunscreens
    II.   external analgesics
    III.   Anti-infectives

    a.   I only
    b.   III only
    c.   I and II only
    d.   II and III only
    e.   I, II, and III

NAPLEX SAMPLE EXAMINATION KEY

1	c	11	c	21	a	31	d	41	a	51	a	61	e	71	c	81	b	91	d
2	c	12	b	22	a	32	a	42	e	52	b	62	a	72	c	82	e	92	a
3	d	13	d	23	c	33	a	43	b	53	c	63	a	73	a	83	e	93	e
4	a	14	e	24	c	34	b	44	a	54	d	64	c	74	c	84	c	94	e
5	a	15	c	25	d	35	d	45	b	55	b	65	e	75	a	85	c	95	b
6	a	16	c	26	e	36	a	46	b	56	e	66	c	76	b	86	a	96	e
7	b	17	c	27	c	37	d	47	e	57	c	67	d	77	b	87	e	97	c
8	a	18	a	28	b	38	b	48	d	58	e	68	d	78	a´	88	c	98	d
9	b	19	a	29	c	39	b	49	a	59	e	69	c	79	b	89	b	99	e
10	a	20	e	30	b	40	b	50	c	60	e	70	b	80	b	90	b	100	c

BIBLIOGRAPHY

1.   1996-1997 NAPLEX Candidate's Review Guide, National Association of Boards of Pharmacy, Park Ridge, Illinois 60068; 1995.

2.   Handbook of Nonprescription Drugs, American Pharmaceutical Association (APhA), Washington, DC 20037; 1996.

3.   DiGregorio GJ, Barbieri EJ. Handbook of Commonly Prescribed Drugs, 6th Edition 1991.

4.   Noah R. Certification Review For Pharmacy Technicians, 2nd Edition 1996.

5.   Manning GW. Handbook of Over-The-Counter Products 1992.

6.   Lloyd YY, Koda-Kimble MA (eds). Applied Therapeutics: The Clinical Use of Drugs, 4th Edition 1988;1663-1742; P.O. Box 5077, Vancouver, WA 98668.

7.   Facts and Comparisons, Facts and Comparisons, Inc. St.Louis, MO 63146-3098.

8.   Albert MB, Callaway CW. Clinical Nutrition for the House Officer 1992. Williams & Wilkins, Baltimore, MD 21202.

9.   Remington's Pharmaceutical Sciences, 17th Edition, 1985; Mack Printing Company, Easton, Pennsylvania, PA.

10.   *U.S. Pharmacist* 1996;21(6):122-123.

11.   Tyler VE. Herbs of Choice: The Therapeutic Use of Phytomedicinals 1994. Pharmaceutical Products Press, Inc., 10 Alice Street, Binghamton, NY 13904-1580.

12.   Micky S. *Drug Topics* 1996 (January 22).

APPENDIX I

Medications Proposed For OTC Status or Recently Obtaining OTC Status.

Dermatologic Agents	Gastrointestinal Agents	Genitourinary Agents	Musculoskeletal Agents	Ophthalmic Agents
Acyclovir Erythromycin Tretinoin Chlortetracycline	Dicyclomine **H$_2$-antagonists:** *Cimetidine* *Famotidine* *Ranitidine* *Nizatidine* Metoclopramide Promethazine suppository Trimethobenzamide **Proton Pump Inhibitor** Omeprazole (Prilosec)	Oral contraceptives **Antifungals:** Butoconazole Nystatin Terconazole *Ticonazole* *Miconazole* *Clotrimazole* Fluconazole Methenamine Phenazopyridine	**NSAIDS:** *Ibuprofen* Diflunisal Fenoprofen *Ketoprofen* *Naproxen sodium* Tolmetin **Topical NSAIDS:** Diclofenac Ketoprofen Ibuprofen Piroxicam Felbinac **Muscle Relaxants:** Cyclobenzaprine Chlorzoxazone Methocarbamol	Chloramphenicol Cromolyn sodium Oxybuprocaine
Respiratory Agents	**Central Nervous System Agents**	**Cardiovascular Agents**	**Cholesterol-Lowering Agents**	**Miscellaneous**
Cromolyn sodium Select nonsedating antihistamines *Select sedating antihistamines* Inhaled topical corticosteroids	Beta-blockers Temazepam Sumatriptan *Nicotine replacement agents*	Erythrityl tetranitrate Nitroglycerine	Cholestyramine Colestipol HMG-Co-A reductase inhibitors	*Minoxidil topical* Hyoscine patch Erythromycin (systemic)

Mickey S. Drug Topics 1996 (January 22). Note: Those products that have been granted Rx-to-OTC conversion are italicized.

APPENDIX II

Safe Use Of
Over-The-Counter (OTC) Medicines

Access + Knowledge = Power

- American medicine cabinets contain a growing choice of OTC medicines to treat an expanding range of ailments.
- OTC medicines often do more than relieve aches, pains and itches.
- Some can prevent diseases like tooth decay, cure diseases like athletes foot and, with a doctor's guidance, help manage chronic and recurring conditions from vaginitis to arthritis.
- The U.S. Food and Drug Administration (FDA) determines whether medicines are prescription or nonprescription.
- The term prescription (Rx) refers to medicines that are safe and effective when used under a doctor's order.
- Nonprescription (OTC) drugs are medicines FDA decides are safe and effective for use without a doctor's prescription.
- FDA also decides when a prescription drug is safe enough to be sold directly to consumers over the counter.
- The regulatory process allowing Americans to take a more active role in their care is known as Rx-to-OTC switch.
- As a result of this process, more than 600 products sold over the counter today use ingredients or dosage strengths available only by prescription 20 years ago.
- Increased access to OTC medicines is especially important for our maturing population.
- Two out of three older Americans rate their health as excellent to good, but four out of five report at least one chronic condition. (For example, almost half of all persons 65 and older have arthritis.)
- Fact is, today's nonprescription medicines offer greater opportunity to treat more of the aches and illnesses most likely to appear in our later years. As we live longer, work longer and take more active role in our own health care, the need grows to become better informed about self-care.
- The best way to become better informed-for young and old alike-is to read and understand the information on OTC labels.
- Next to the medicine itself, it's the most important part of self-care with nonprescription medicines.
- With new opportunities in self-medication come new responsibilities and a growing need for knowledge.

Source: Nonprescription Drug Manufacturers Association (NDMA)
(Reprinted with permission)

It's On The Label

- A description of tamper-resistant feature(s) to check before you buy the product
- The product name
- Ingredients - Active & Inactive
- Any recent significant product changes
- Indications - What the medicine is for
- "Usual Dosage" - Directions for use
- "Warnings" - When to stop taking the medicine; when to see a doctor; possible side effects
- "Expiration Date" - When to throw it out

OTC Know-How Is On The Label

- You wouldn't ignore your doctor's instructions for using a prescription drug; so don't ignore the label when taking a nonprescription medicine.
- Some medicines, though, come in small packages-and reading the label is not always easy.
- That's why the OTC industry and FDA are working to make medicine labels easier to read-and easier to understand.
- You can help yourself too. Always use enough light (it usually takes three times more light to read the same line at age 60 than at age 30) and use your glasses or contact lenses when reading labels!
- When it comes to medicines, more does not necessarily mean better. You should never misuse OTC medicines by taking them longer or in higher doses than the label recommends. Symptoms that persist are a clear signal it's time to see a doctor.
- Remember, if you read the label and still have questions, talk to a doctor, nurse or pharmacist.

Drug Interactions: A Word To The Wise

- Although mild and relatively uncommon, interactions involving OTC drugs can produce unwanted results or make medicines less effective.
- It's especially important to know about drug interactions if you're taking Rx and OTC drugs at the same time.
- Some drugs can also interact with foods and beverages, as well as with health conditions such as diabetes, kidney disease and high blood pressure.
- Here are a few drug interaction cautions for some common OTC ingredients:
- Avoid alcohol if you are taking antihistamines, cough-cold products with the ingredient dextromethorphan or drugs that treat sleeplessness (Sleep Aids/CNS Stimulants/ Cough&Cold - Tables).
- Do not use drugs that treat sleeplessness if you are taking prescription sedatives or tranquilizers (Benzodiazepines).
- Check with your doctor or pharmacist before taking products containing aspirin if you're taking a prescription blood thinner or if you have diabetes or gout (UA).
- Do not use laxatives (Table) when you have stomach pain, nausea or vomiting.
- Do not use cough-cold or weight-control medicines (Table) with the ingredient phenyl-

propanolamine (PPA) if you're being treated for high blood pressure or depression (MAOIs), or if you have heart disease, diabetes or thyroid disease (Incr. metabolism).

- Unless directed by a doctor, do not use a nasal decongestant (sympathomimetics) if you are taking a prescription drug for high blood pressure or depression, or if you have heart or thyroid disease, diabetes or prostate problems.
- This is not a complete list. Read the label! Drug labels change as new information becomes available. That's why it's important to read the label each time you take medicine.

Time For A Medicine Cabinet Checkup?
- Be sure to look through your medicine supply at least once a year.
- Always store medicines in a cool, dry place (change in integrity).
- Discard any medicines that are past the expiration date (Brown bag).
- To make sure no one takes the wrong medicine, keep all medicines in their original containers.

Pregnancy And Nursing
- Drugs can pass from a pregnant woman to her unborn baby. A safe concentration of medicine for the mother may be a high concentration for the baby. If you're pregnant, always talk with your doctor or pharmacist before taking any drugs, Rx or OTC.
  (Table - Drugs safe in pregnancy & lactation)
- Although most drugs pass into breast milk in concentrations too low to have any unwanted effects on the baby, breast-feeding mothers still need to be careful.
- A doctor or pharmacist can tell you how to adjust the timing and dosing of most medicines so the baby is exposed to the lowest amount possible.
- Some drugs should be avoided altogether. Always ask your doctor or pharmacist before taking any medicine while breast-feeding.

Kids Aren't Just Small Adults
- OTC drugs rarely come in one-size-fits-all. Here are some tips about giving OTC medicines to children:
- Children aren't just small adults, so don't estimate the dose based on their size. Read the label.
- Know the difference between TBSP. (tablespoon = 15 mL) and TSP.   (teaspoon = 5 mL). They are very different doses.
- Be careful about converting dose instructions. If the label says two teaspoons, it's best to use a measuring spoon or a dosing cup marked in teaspoons.
- Don't play doctor. Don't double the dose just because your child seems sicker than last time. (Give a dose a chance to work!)
- Before you give your child two medicines at the same time, talk to your doctor or pharmacist.
- Follow any age limits on the label.
- Never let children take medicine by themselves.
- Never describe medicine as candy to get your kids to take it. If they come across the medicine on their own, they're likely to remember that you called it candy.

Child-Resistant Packaging

- Child-resistant caps are designed for repeated use to make it difficult for children to open. Remember, if you don't re-lock the cap after each use, the child-resistant device can't do its job - keeping children out!
- It's best to store all medicines - including vitamins and supplements - where children can neither see nor reach them.
- Containers of pills should not be left on the kitchen counter as a reminder.
- Purses and briefcases are among the worst places to hide drugs from curious kids.
- And since are natural mimics, it's a good idea not to take medicine in front of them. They are tempted to "play house" with your medicine later on.
- Be especially careful with iron-containing supplements. Iron is the leading cause of fatal ingestion poisonings (Iron Overload!) in children under three.
- If you find some packages too difficult to open - and don't have young children living with you or visiting - you should know the law allows one package size for each medicine to be sold without child-resistant features. If you don't see it on the store shelf, ask.

(Musculoskeletal Diseases - Must document and have customer sign)

Protect Yourself Against Tampering

- Makers of OTC medicines seal most products in tamper-resistant packaging (TRP) to help protect against criminal tampering.
- TRP works by providing visible evidence if the the package has been disturbed.
- But OTC packaging cannot be 100 percent tamper-proof.
- Here is how to help protect yourseif:
- Be alert to the tamper-resistant features on the package before you open it. These features are described on the label.
- Inspect the outer packaging before you buy it. When you get home, inspect the medicine inside.
- Don't buy an OTC product if the packaging is damaged.
- Don't use any medicine that looks discolored or different in any way.
- If anything looks suspicious, be suspicious. Contact the store where you bought the product. Take it back!
- Never take medicines in the dark.   (NDMA – Reprinted with permission)

Note: Page numbers followed by *t* and *f* denote tables and figures, respectively.

anorexia, 77*t*

anorexiants, 23*t*–24*t*

antacids, 27*t*–29*t*. *See also specific drug*
    case scenario, 104
    composition and acid neutralizing capacity, 29*t*
    drug interactions, 28*t*

antibiotics, first-aid, 98*t*

anticancer herbs, 91*t*–92*t*

anticholinergics, gastrointestinal, 30*t*–31*t*

antidiarrheals, 30*t*–31*t*, 76*t*

antiemetics, 35*t*

antiflatulents, 27*t*

antifungal powders, 70*t*

antihistamines. *See also specific drug*
    in cold/cough/allergy products, 36*t*
    drug interactions, 38*t*
    non-sedating, 38*t*
    for prevention of motion sickness, 35*t*
    side effects of, 36*t*
    for sleep management, 21*t*

anti-infective herbs, 78*t*

antimigraine herbs, 84*t*

antipyretics, 25*t*–26*t*

antiseptics
    first-aid, 97*t*
    herbal, 77*t*

antitussives, 36*t*
    demulcent, 79*t*
    side effects of, 36*t*

anti-ulcer combinations, 28*t*

Antivert. *See* meclizine hydrochloride

Anucort-HC. *See* hydrocortisone acetate

Anusol H. *See* pramoxine

Anusol-HC. *See* hydrocortisone acetate; hydrocortisone cream

anxiety disorders, 83*t*

APAP, 37*t*

aphrodisiacs, 84*t*

APIGARD. *See* polyurethane foam dressings

apocynum, 82*t*

appetite loss, 23*t*–24*t*, 77*t*

appetite stimulants, 24*t*

appetite suppressants, 23*t*

apricot, 92*t*

aquaretic herbs, 77*t*

Aquasol A. *See* vitamin A (beta carotene)

Aquasol E. *See* vitamin E (tocopherol)
Arctostaphylos uva-ursi. See uva-ursi
arnica, 86*t*
arsenic, 93*t*
arteriosclerosis, 81*t*
ArthiCare Ultra. *See* capsaicin, and menthol
arthritis, 86*t*–87*t*, 89*t*
ascorbic acid (vitamin C), 41*t*
    and iron, 46*t*
Ascorbicap. *See* ascorbic acid (vitamin C)
Ascriptin. *See* aspirin
Ascriptin A/D. *See* aspirin
ashwangandha, 90*t*
aspirin, 25*t*
    with acetaminophen and caffeine, 25*t*
assessment, patient, 19
Astelin. *See* azelastine
astemizole, 38*t*
asthma, 61*t*
asthma, bronchial, 79*t*
astringents, for hemorrhoids, 34*t*
athlete's foot, 70*t*
atopic dermatitis, 68*t*
Atrocol Elixir, 31*t*
atropine, intranasal, 38*t*
atropine sulfate, 26*t*, 30*t*–31*t*
Atrovent. *See* ipratropium bromide
attapulgite, 30*t*
Attend, 72*t*
Aueromycin. *See* chlortetracycline 3% ointment
Aveeno Colloidal Oatmeal, 66*t*
Axid AR. *See* nizatidine
azatadine, 38*t*
azelastine, 36*t*
Azo-Gantanol. *See* sulfamethoxazole, and phenazopyridine hydrochloride
Azo-Gantrisin. *See* sulfisoxazole, and phenazopyridine hydrochloride
Azo-Standard. *See* phenazopyridine hydrochloride

B
Baciguent, 98*t*
bacitracin, 98*t*
Bactine First-Aid, 98*t*
baking soda, 27*t*, 70*t*
basil, 88*t*
Bausch & Lomb Allergy Drops. *See* naphazoline hydrochloride

Bayer. *See* aspirin
Bayer Select MS. *See* diphenhydramine
bearberry, 77t
beclomethasone, 38t
bee stings, 66t
belladonna alkaloids, 30t
belladonna extract, plus butabarbital and alcohol, 31t
Benadryl. *See* diphenhydramine
Benadryl Allergy Decongestant, 37t
Ben-Gay. *See* menthol; methyl salicylate
Benylin Multisymptom, 37t
benzalkonium chloride, 97t
benzene, 94t
benzethonium chloride, 97t
benzocaine, 23t, 34t, 65t–66t
benzoic acid, 26t
benzoyl peroxide, 66t
benzphetamine hydrochloride, 24t
benzyl alcohol, 65t
beta-carotene (vitamin A), 40t
Betadine. *See* povidone-iodine complex
Betadine Douche, 63t
bilberries, 76t
BioBrane II. *See* biosynthetic dressings
biosynthetic dressings, 99t
birch leaves, 77t
bisacodyl, 32t
Bismatrol. *See* bismuth salts (bismuth subsalicylate)
Bismatrol Extra Strength. *See* bismuth salts (bismuth subsalicylate)
bismuth salts (bismuth subsalicylate), 27t, 30t
    plus metronidazole and tetracycline, 28t
bitter herbs, 77t
bitterstick, 77t
blackberry leaves, 76t
blackberry root, 76t
black cohosh, 85t
black currant, 85t
black hellebore, 82t
black indian hemp, 82t
blessed thistle, 77t
Blinx, 59t
blood glucose reagent strips, 56t
blood glucose reflectance meters, 55t
blood glucose test products, 51t
blood pressure monitoring devices, home, 61t

bloodroot, 88*t*
blood stain removal, 61*t*
blueberries, 76*t*
blueberry leaves, 76*t*
bogbean, 77*t*
boldo, 75*t*
Bonine. *See* meclizine hydrochloride
Bontril PDM. *See* phendimetrazine tartrate
borage seed, 85*t*
breastfeeding, OTC medications during, 16, 49*t*, 139
bromodiphenhydramine, 37*t*
brompheniramine maleate, 36*t*–37*t*
bronchial asthma, 79*t*
BSS. *See* bismuth salts (bismuth subsalicylate)
buckthorn bark, 74*t*
Bufferin. *See* aspirin
Bufferin AF Nite Time Caplets. *See* diphenhydramine
Bufferin Arthritis Strength. *See* aspirin
buffers, ocular, 59*t*
bugle weed, 85*t*
bulk producers, for weight control, 23*t*
bulk-producing laxatives, 32*t*–33*t*
bupropion hydrochloride, 95*t*
burns, 86*t*
Burow's solution. *See* aluminum acetate
butabarbital, plus belladonna extract and alcohol, 31*t*
butcher's-broom, 82*t*
Butibel Elixir. *See* butabarbital, plus belladonna extract and alcohol
butoconazole nitrate, 63*t*

C

cacao (cocoa), 20*t*, 84*t*
cactus grandiflorus, 82*t*
Caffedrine. *See* caffeine
caffeine, 20*t*, 90*t*
       with aspirin and acetaminophen, 25*t*
       in beverages, 84*t*
       in cough/cold/allergy products, 37*t*
       in non-pharmacologic products, 20*t*, 84*t*
       in pharmacologic products, 20*t*
       in plants, 84*t*
calamine, 34*t*, 66*t*
Cal Carb-HD. *See* calcium
Calci-Chew. *See* calcium
Calciday. *See* calcium

drug review, FDA advisory panels for, 10
drug storage, patient counseling about, 139
Dry Eyes, 59*t*
dry mouth, 36*t*
dry powder inhalers, 61*t*
DSS. *See* docusate sodium
Dulcolax. *See* bisacodyl
Dull-C. *See* ascorbic acid (vitamin C)
duodenal ulcers, 28*t*, 76*t*
Duplex T. *See* coal tar shampoo
Duration. *See* oxymetazoline hydrochloride
dyclonine, 65*t*
dyspepsia, 27*t*–29*t*, 75*t*

E

Ear Drops, 60*t*
Ear Drops by Murine, 60*t*
ear plugs, 60*t*
ear wax, 60*t*
Easpirin. *See* aspirin
echinacea, 91*t*
E-Complex. *See* vitamin E (tocopherol)
Ecotrin. *See* aspirin
eczema, 68*t*
Efidac. *See* pseudoephedrine
E-400 I.U. Capsules. *See* vitamin E (tocopherol)
E-200 I.U. Softgels. *See* vitamin E (tocopherol)
E-1000 I.U. Softgels. *See* vitamin E (tocopherol)
ElastoGel. *See* hydrogels/gels
electrolyte imbalance, pediatric formulas to correct, 49*t*
eleuthero, 90*t*
emetics, 35*t*
Emetrol. *See* phosphorated carbohydrate
emollients, 32*t*–33*t*
Empirin. *See* aspirin
Emulsoil. *See* castor oil
Encare, 62*t*
Endal. *See* phenylephrine hydrochloride
endocrine disorders, 85*t*
endurance enhancers, 90*t*
enemas, laxative, 32*t*
Ener-B. *See* vitamin B_{12} (cyanocobalamin)
Enfamil, 49*t*
Enfamil Premature Formula, 49*t*
English walnut leaves, 86*t*

G

garlic, 81*t*
gastric ulcers, 28*t*, 76*t*
gastrointestinal disorders, 74*t*–77*t*
gauze dressings, 99*t*
Gelusil, 29*t*. *See also* magnesium and aluminum combinations
Gelusil-II, 29*t*
Gencalc 600. *See* calcium
generic drugs, 15
Genlax-S. *See* docusate sodium, and senna
gentian, 77*t*
Gevral Protein, 50*t*
ginger, 74*t*, 76*t*
gingival disorders, 86*t*
ginkgo, 81*t*, 84*t*
ginseng, 90*t*
glucagon, 51*t*
Glucometer II, 55*t*
Glucometer M, 55*t*
glucometers, 51*t*, 55*t*
Glucoscan, 55*t*
Glucoscan strips, 55*t*
Glucoscan 3000 with Memory, 55*t*
glucose oxidase methods, of glucose testing, 57*t*
glucose reagent strips, blood, 56*t*
glucose reflectance meters, blood, 55*t*
glucose tests
   blood, 51*t*, 55*t*
   urine, 51*t*, 57*t*
      drug interference with, 58*t*
Glucostix, 56*t*
Glucostrix, 55*t*
glycerin, anhydrous, in isopropyl alcohol, 60*t*
glycerin suppositories, 33*t*
glycosides, cardioactive, 82*t*
Glycyrrhiza. *See* licorice
golden rod, 77*t*
goldenseal, 88*t*
gotu kola, 62
grapeseed, 82*t*
guaifenesin, 36*t*–37*t*
Guaituss. *See* guaifenesin
guarana, 84*t*
guggul, 88*t*
gynecological disorders, 85*t*

Gyne-Lotrimin Vaginal Inserts. *See* clotrimazole
Gynol, 62*t*

H

hair regrowth products, 66*t*
Haltran. *See* ibuprofen
hamamelis water, 34*t*, 86*t*
H$_2$ antagonists, 28*t*
hawthorn, 62, 81*t*
headache, 84*t*
head lice, 66*t*
Head & Shoulders. *See* pyrithione zinc shampoo; selenium sulfide shampoo
health supplies, 61*t*
Helidac. *See* metronidazole, plus tetracycline and bismuth subsalicylate
Hemaspan. *See* iron
Hemorrhoidal-HC. *See* hydrocortisone acetate
hemorrhoidals, 34*t*
Hemril-HC Uniserts. *See* hydrocortisone acetate
Hepatic-Aid, 50*t*
hepatotoxicity, 76*t*
herbs, 74*t*–92*t*. *See also specific herb*
        case scenario, 107
hexylresorcinol, 65*t*, 97*t*
Hismanal. *See* astemizole
HIV detection kit, home, 61*t*
Home Access, 61*t*
home diagnostic test kits, 61*t*
hops, 83*t*
horehound, 80*t*
horse chestnut seed, 82*t*
Humibid. *See* guaifenesin
humidifiers, 61*t*
Hycotuss Expectorant, 37*t*
Hydragran. *See* exudate absorbers
Hydrastis canadensis. *See* goldenseal
Hydrocii Instant. *See* psyllium
hydrocodone, 37*t*
hydrocolloids, 99*t*
hydrocortisone, 68*t*
hydrocortisone acetate, 34*t*
hydrocortisone cream, 34*t*
hydrogels/gels, 99*t*
hydrogen cyanide, 93*t*
hydrogen peroxide, 97*t*
hygiene, personal, 63*t*

hyoscyamine, 26*t*, 30*t*–31*t*
Hypericum perforatum. See St. John's wort
hyperthyroidism, 85*t*
hypodermic equipment, 51*t*, 61*t*
Hytuss. *See* guaifenesin

I

ibuprofen, 25*t*, 63*t*
Iceland moss, 79*t*
identification tags, for diabetics, 51*t*
Ilex paraguariensis. See maté
imidazolidinyl urea, 63*t*
immunotherapy, 91*t*
Imodium. *See* loperamide
Imodium AD. *See* loperamide
impotence, sexual, 84*t*
indigestion, 27*t*–29*t*, 75*t*
infant formulas, 49*t*
infectious disease, 77*t*–78*t*, 86*t*, 91*t*. *See also specific disease*
Inhal-Aid, 61*t*
inhalers, 61*t*
insect repellents, 66*t*
insomnia. *See* sleep aids
Inspirease, 61*t*
Instant Breakfast, 50*t*
insulins, 51*t*–54*t*
       intermediate-acting, 53*t*
       long-acting, 54*t*
       short-acting, 52*t*
internal analgesics, 25*t*
       case scenario, 103
interview, patient, 19
Iocon. *See* coal tar shampoo
iodine, 44*t*, 97*t*
Ionamin. *See* phentermine
Ionil. *See* coal tar shampoo
ipecac syrup, 35*t*, 80*t*
ipratropium bromide, 38*t*
iron, 45*t*–46*t*
      and vitamin C, 46*t*
Iron Dextran (InFeD). *See* iron
Ironspan. *See* iron
irrigating solutions, ocular, 59*t*
irritant laxatives, 32*t*–33*t*
Isocal, 50*t*

Isomil, 49*t*
isopropyl alcohol, 97*t*
    anhydrous glycerin in, 60*t*
ivy, 80*t*

J

jewelweed, 86*t*
jock itch, 70*t*
juniper, 77*t*

K

Kaltostat. *See* alginates
Kaodene Non-Narcotic. *See* attapulgite
kaolin-pectin, 30*t*
Kaopectate. *See* attapulgite
Kaopectate II Caplets. *See* loperamide
Kaopectate-MS. *See* attapulgite
Kapectolin. *See* kaolin-pectin
Kasof. *See* docusate potassium
K-C. *See* attapulgite
keratolytic shampoo, 67*t*
Keto-Diastix, 57*t*
ketones, urine test, 57*t*
ketoprofen, 25*t*
kidney disorders, 77*t*–78*t*
King of Hearts Tablets, 20*t*
Kondremul. *See* mineral oil
Konsyl. *See* psyllium
K-Pek. *See* attapulgite
K-Y Jelly, 62*t*

L

labeling
    patient counseling about, 138
    readability of, 13
lactation, OTC medications during, 16, 49*t*, 139
lanolin, 34*t*
laxatives, 32*t*–33*t*, 74*t*
    case scenario, 105
    mechanisms of action, 33*t*
lemon balm, 88*t*
Levsin PB Drops, 31*t*
lice, head, 66*t*
licorice, 76*t*, 80*t*
lily-of-the-valley, 82*t*

liver disorders, 76*t*
lobelia, 80*t*
local anesthetics
    in canker/cold sore products, 65*t*
    for hemorrhoids, 34*t*
Lomotil, 31*t*
Loniten. *See* minoxidil
Lonox, 31*t*
loperamide, 30*t*
loratadine, 38*t*
    and pseudoephedrine, 38*t*
Lotrimin Antifungal-AF. *See* clotrimazole
lovage root, 77*t*
lubricant laxatives, 32*t*
LubriTears, 59*t*
LYOfoam. *See* polyurethane foam dressings
LYOfoam "C" Odor Absorbent Dressing. *See* carbon-impregnated dressings

M

Maalox, 29*t*. *See also* magnesium and aluminum combinations
Maalox Anti-Diarrheal Caplets. *See* loperamide
Maalox-ES, 29*t*
Maalox Plus, 29*t*
Maalox Plus-ES, 29*t*
Maalox-TC, 29*t*
Mag-200. *See* magnesium
magaldrate. *See* Riopan
magnesium, 27*t*, 29*t*, 47*t*
magnesium and aluminum combinations, 27*t*, 29*t*
magnesium citrate, 32*t*
magnesium gluconate, 47*t*
magnesium oxide, 47*t*
magnesium sulfate, 32*t*, 47*t*
magnesium trisilicate, 30*t*
357 Magnum II, 20*t*
Magonate. *See* magnesium
Magonate 500. *See* magnesium
Mag-Ox 400. *See* magnesium
Magtrate 500. *See* magnesium
manganese, 47*t*
manganese sulfate, 47*t*
mango, 88*t*
Marezine. *See* cyclizine
Marinol. *See* dronabinol
Marmine. *See* dimenhydrinate

marshmallow root, 79*t*
Massengill Douche, 63*t*
maté, 84*t*
Maximum Strength Neosporin, 98*t*
MDI. *See* metered dose inhalers
meclizine hydrochloride, 35*t*
medical supplies, 61*t*
Medipren. *See* ibuprofen
Medi-Quick, 98*t*
Megace. *See* megestrol acetate
megavitamins, 48*t*
megestrol acetate, 24*t*
Melaleuca alternifolia. See tea tree oil
melatonin, 22*t*
melissa, 88*t*
menadione (vitamin K$_3$), 42*t*
menfegol, 62*t*
menstrual pain, 63*t*
Menthax piperita. See peppermint
menthol, 25*t*, 65*t*, 89*t*, 97*t*
    and capsaicin, 25*t*
      and methyl salicylate, 25*t*
Meridia. *See* sibutramine
metabolic disorders, 85*t*
Metamucil. *See* psyllium
metered dose inhalers, 61*t*
methenamine, 26*t*
methylbenzethonium chloride, 63*t*, 97*t*
methylcellulose, 32*t*
methylene blue, 26*t*
methyl nicotinate, 25*t*
methyl salicylate, 25*t*, 89*t*, 97*t*
    with capsaicin and menthol, 25*t*
metronidazole, plus tetracycline and bismuth subsalicylate, 28*t*
Micatin. *See* miconazole
miconazole, 63*t*, 70*t*
Midol 200. *See* ibuprofen
migraine, 84*t*
milk allergy, infants with, formulas for, 49*t*
Milk of Magnesia, 29*t*, 32*t*. *See also* magnesium
milk thistle, 76*t*
mineral oil, 32*t*, 34*t*
minerals, 39*t*–48*t*. *See also specific mineral*
minoxidil, 66*t*
mistletoe, 92*t*

Mitrolan. *See* polycarbophil

Mol-Iron with Vitamin C. *See* iron, and vitamin C

molybdenum, 47*t*

MOM. *See* milk of magnesia

Monistat-3, 63*t*

Monistat-7, 63*t*

motion sickness, 35*t*, 74*t*

Motrin. *See* ibuprofen

Motrin IB. *See* ibuprofen

mouth, dry, 36*t*

mouth care, 64*t*–65*t*

mouthwashes, 64*t*

MS Dex-A-Diet. *See* phenylpropanolamine

MS Dexatrim. *See* phenylpropanolamine

MS Nytol. *See* diphenhydramine

MS Unisom. *See* diphenhydramine

mucous membrane disorders, 86*t*

mullein flowers, 79*t*

multivitamins, 24*t*

      indications for, 39*t*

Murine Ear Wax Removal Systems, 60*t*

Murine Plus. *See* tetrahydrolozine

musculoskeletal disorders, 86*t*–87*t*, 89*t*

mustard oil, volatile, 89*t*

Mycelex Solution. *See* clotrimazole

Myciguent, 98*t*

Mycitracin Triple Antibiotic, 98*t*

Mylanta, 29*t*. *See also* magnesium and aluminum combinations

Mylanta AR. *See* famotidine

Mylanta-II, 29*t*

Mylicon. *See* simethicone

myrrh, 88*t*

N

NABPLEX. *See under* NAPLEX

Naldecon. *See* guaifenesin

Naldecon-CX, 37*t*

naphazoline hydrochloride, 59*t*

      and pheniramine maleate, 59*t*

naphthalene, 93*t*

NAPLEX competency statements, 5–7

NAPLEX review examination, sample, 112–134

naproxen, 25*t*

Nasalcrom. *See* cromolyn sodium

Nature's Remedy. *See* aloes, with cascara sagrada

nausea, 35*t*, 74*t*

N.B.P., 98*t*

nebulizers, 61*t*

neem, 88*t*

Neo-Calgucon. *See* calcium

Neomixin, 98*t*

neomycin, 98*t*

Neosporin, 98*t*

Neo-Synephrine. *See* phenylephrine hydrochloride

Nephro-Calci. *See* calcium

Nervine. *See* diphenhydramine

nervous system disorders, 83*t*–84*t*

Nestrex. *See* vitamin B$_6$ (pyridoxine)

Neutragena T/Gel. *See* coal tar shampoo

Neutra-Phos-K Capsules. *See* calcium phosphate

Neutra-Phos-K Powder. *See* calcium phosphate

Neutra-Phos Powder. *See* calcium phosphate

Neutrogena. *See* benzoyl peroxide

Nia-Bid. *See* vitamin B$_3$ (niacin)

Niac. *See* vitamin B$_3$ (niacin)

Niacels. *See* vitamin B$_3$ (niacin)

niacin (vitamin B$_3$), 40*t*

NicCheck I, 61*t*, 95*t*

N'ice Vitamin C Drops, 41*t*

Nico-400. *See* vitamin B$_3$ (niacin)

Nicobid Tempules. *See* vitamin B$_3$ (niacin)

Nicoderm. *See* nicotine transdermal systems

NicoDerm CQ. *See* nicotine patch

Nicorette. *See* nicotine polacrilex gum

nicotine, 94*t*

nicotine & byproducts test, urine, 61*t*

nicotine nasal spray, 95*t*

nicotine patch, 95*t*

nicotine polacrilex gum, 95*t*

nicotine transdermal systems, 95*t*–96*t*

     advantages over other nicotine products, 96*t*

Nicotinex. *See* vitamin B$_3$ (niacin)

nicotinic acid. *See* vitamin B$_3$ (niacin)

Nicotrol. *See* nicotine transdermal systems

Nicotrol Inhaler, 95*t*

Nicotrol NS. *See* nicotine nasal spray

Niferex with Vitamin C. *See* iron, and vitamin C

Nighttime Pamprin. *See* diphenhydramine

Nix. *See* permethril

nizatidine, 28*t*

patient interview, 19

pau d'arco, 92*t*

Paulinia cupana. See guarana

Pazos & Wyanoids hemorrhoidal suppositories, 34*t*

peak expiratory flow rate (PEFR) meters, 61*t*

Pedialyte Imbalance, 49*t*

Pedialyte RS, 49*t*

pediatric patients, guidelines for, 139–140

Pentrax. *See* coal tar shampoo

Pep-Back Tablets, 20*t*

Pep-Back Ultra Caplets, 20*t*

Pepcid AC. *See* famotidine

peppermint, 75*t*

peptic ulcers, 28*t*, 76*t*

Pepto-Bismol. *See* bismuth salts (bismuth subsalicylate)

Pepto-Bismol Maximum Strength. *See* bismuth salts (bismuth subsalicylate)

Pepto Diarrhea Control. *See* loperamide

performance enhancers, 90*t*

Periactin. *See* cyproheptadine hydrochloride

Peri-Colace. *See* casanthranol, and docusate sodium

peripheral vascular disease, 81*t*–82*t*

permethril, 66*t*

personal care products, 63*t*

petrolatum, 34*t*

pharmaceutical care, comprehensive, 18–19

pharmacist-patient consultation process. *See* patient counseling

phenazopyridine hydrochloride, 26*t*

    plus sulfamethizole and oxytetracycline hydrochloride, 26*t*

    and sulfamethoxazole, 26*t*

    and sulfisoxazole, 26*t*

phendimetrazine tartrate, 24*t*

pheniramine maleate, and naphazoline hydrochloride, 59*t*

phenobarbital, 31*t*

phenol, 64*t*–65*t*, 97*t*

phenolate sodium, 65*t*

phenolphthalein, 32*t*

    and docusate sodium, 32*t*

Phenoxine. *See* phenylpropanolamine

phentermine hydrochloride, 24*t*

phenylephrine hydrochloride, 34*t*, 36*t*–37*t*, 59*t*

phenylpropanolamine, 23*t*, 36*t*–37*t*

phenyl salicylate, 26*t*

Phillips MOM. *See* milk of magnesia

Phos-Ex. *See* calcium

phosphate compounds, 32*t*

protein, high, infant formulas with, 49*t*
pseudoephedrine, 36*t*–37*t*
    and fexofenadine, 38*t*
    and loratadine, 38*t*
    and terfenadine, 38*t*
psyllium, 32*t*
Pulmocare, 50*t*
Puralube Tears, 59*t*
Purge. *See* castor oil
Pyridium. *See* phenazopyridine hydrochloride
pyridoxine hydrochloride (vitamin B$_6$), 40*t*
pyrilamine maleate, 21*t*
pyrithione zinc shampoo, 67*t*–68*t*

Q
Quick-Pep. *See* caffeine

R
radioactive compounds, in cigarette smoke, 93*t*
ranitidine, 28*t*
ranitidine bismuth citrate, and clarithromycin, 28*t*
ranitidine hydrochloride, 28*t*
raspberry leaves, 76*t*, 85*t*
Redux. *See* dexfenfluramine
refrigerants, 89*t*
Reguloid. *See* psyllium
Reliance, 73*t*
respiratory therapy instruments, 61*t*
respiratory tract disorders, 79*t*–80*t*
Retinol. *See* vitamin A (beta carotene)
Retinol-A. *See* vitamin A (beta carotene)
Rexigen Forte SR. *See* phendimetrazine tartrate
rhatany, 88*t*
Rheaban-MS. *See* attapulgite
rhubarb, 74*t*
Ribes nigrum. *See* black currant
riboflavin (vitamin B$_2$), 40*t*
Rid-A-Pain. *See* methyl nicotinate
Riopan, 29*t*
Riopan-ES, 29*t*
Riopan Plus, 29*t*
Riopan Plus 2, 29*t*
Robitussin. *See* guaifenesin
Robitussin A-C. *See* guaifenesin
Robitussin-CF. *See* guaifenesin

Robitussin-DM. *See* guaifenesin
Rogaine. *See* minoxidil
Rogaine ES. *See* minoxidil
Rolaids. *See* calcium carbonate
Rondec-DM, 37*t*
rosemary, 82*t*
rubefacients, 89*t*
Rufen. *See* ibuprofen

S

sabal. *See* saw palmetto
sage, 88*t*
salicyl alcohol, 65*t*
salicylic acid, 67*t*, 70*t*
saline laxatives, 32*t*–33*t*
saliva, artificial, 36*t*
saliva substitutes, 36*t*
Salix alba. See willow bark
sample OTC Naplex review examination, 112–133
Sani-Supp. *See* glycerin suppositories
sanitary napkins, 63*t*
sarsaparilla, 90*t*
sassafras, 90*t*
saw palmetto, 78*t*
schizandra, 76*t*
scopolamine, 31*t*
Scott's Emulsion, 50*t*
seborrheic dermatitis, 68*t*
Sebulon. *See* pyrithione zinc shampoo
Seldane. *See* terfenadine
Seldane-D. *See* terfenadine, and pseudoephedrine
selenium, 48*t*
selenium sulfide shampoo, 67*t*–68*t*
Selsun Blue. *See* selenium sulfide shampoo
Semicid, 62*t*
senega snakeroot, 80*t*
Senexon. *See* senna
senna, 32*t*, 74*t*
        and docusate sodium, 32*t*
Senokot. *See* senna
Senokot-S. *See* docusate sodium, and senna
Senolax. *See* senna
Septa, 98*t*
Serenoa repens. See saw palmetto
Serostim. *See* somatropin

Z

Zantac 75. *See* ranitidine
Zantac 75 EFFERdose. *See* ranitidine hydrochloride
Zetar. *See* coal tar shampoo
zinc, 48*t*
Zinc-220. *See* zinc sulfate
Zincate. *See* zinc sulfate
zinc gluconate, 48*t*
Zincon. *See* pyrithione zinc shampoo
zinc sulfate, 48*t*
zinc undecylenate, 70*t*
Zingiber officinale. See ginger
ZNP Bar. *See* pyrithione zinc shampoo
Zostrix, 83*t. See* capsaicin cream
Zostrix-HP. *See* capsaicin cream
Zyban. *See* bupropion hydrochloride
Zyrtec. *See* cetirizine